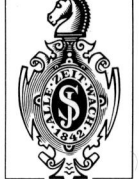

J. Brachmann R. Dietz W. Kübler (Eds.)

Heart Failure and Arrhythmias

With 41 Figures and 17 Tables

Springer-Verlag
Berlin Heidelberg New York
London Paris Tokyo
Hong Kong Barcelona

Priv.-Doz. JOHANNES BRACHMANN, MD
Prof. RAINER DIETZ, MD
Prof. WOLFGANG KÜBLER, MD
Department of Internal Medicine III, Cardiology
Medizinische Universitätsklinik
Bergheimer Str. 58
6900 Heidelberg, FRG

ISBN 3-540-52041-4 Springer-Verlag Berlin Heidelberg New York
ISBN 0-387-52041-4 Springer-Verlag New York Berlin Heidelberg

Library of Congress Cataloging-in-Publication Data. Heart failure and arrhythmias / J. Brachmann, R. Dietz, W. Kübler, (eds.). p. cm. Based on an international satellite workshop to the World Congress of Clinical Pharmacology, held in Heidelberg/Mannheim from July 23–29, 1989. Includes bibliographical references. Includes index.
ISBN 3-540-52041-4 (Berlin). – ISBN 0-387-52041-4 (New York)
1. Congestive heart failure–Congresses. 2. Heart failure–Congresses. 3. Arrhythmia–Congresses. I. Brachmann, J. II. Dietz, R. (Rainer). III. Kübler, W. IV. World Congress of Clinical Pharmacology (1989: Heidelberg, Germany and Mannheim, Germany) [DNLM: 1. Arrhythmia–drug therapy–congresses. 2. Arrhythmia-physiopathology–congresses. 3. Heart Failure, Congestive–drug therapy–congresses. 4. Heart Failure, Congestive–physiopathology-congresses. WG 370 H4362 1989] RC685.C53H43 1990 616.1'2–dc20 DNLM/DLC for Library of Congress 90-9813 CIP.

This work is subject to copyright. All rights are reserved, whether the whole or part of the material is concerned, specifically the rights of translation, reprinting, reuse of illustrations, recitation, broadcasting, reproduction on microfilms or in other ways, and storage in data banks. Duplication of this publication or parts thereof is only permitted under the provisions of the German Copyright Law of September 9, 1965, in its current version, and a copyright fee must always be paid. Violations fall under the prosecution act of the German Copyright Law.

© Springer-Verlag Berlin Heidelberg 1990
Printed in Germany

The use of registered names, trademarks, etc. in this publication does not imply, even in the absence of a specific statement, that such names are exempt from the relevant protective laws and regulations and therefore free for general use.

Product Liability: The publishers can give no guarantee for information about drug dosage and application thereof contained in this book. In every individual case the respective user must check its accuracy by consulting other pharmaceutical literature.

Typesetting, printing and bookbinding:
Konrad Triltsch, Graphischer Betrieb, 8700 Würzburg, FRG
2119/3130-543210 – Printed on acid-free paper

Preface

Heart failure is a clinical entity characterized by a certain combination of symptoms and signs. Although there is neither a definition covering all aspects of it nor any generally accepted criteria for evaluating its severity, it is the endstage of many different heart diseases, in most cases associated with a poor prognosis. Approximately 50% of the patients with advanced heart failure die from pump failure, whereas the other half succumb suddenly and unexpectedly due to ventricular tachyarrhythmias. Although impaired left ventricular function is the main risk factor, sudden death may already occur in less severe cases of heart failure. In certain cardiac diseases, such as dilative cardiomyopathy, the occurrence of ventricular arrhythmias may be related directly to the underlying heart disease, as the frequency and severity (Lown classification) of ventricular ectopics are not related to left ventricular impairment.

Treatment of ventricular tachyarrhythmias is still an unsolved problem, especially in patients with heart failure, who need it the most. The vast majority of antiarrhythmic agents are more or less negatively inotropic and may therefore substantially aggravate ventricular impairment. Nonpharmacological approaches – such as the implantation of a defibrillator – still require major surgery with the associated increased risk to the patient in heart failure.

No agreement has yet been reached on the criteria for evaluating how effective treatment has been, either for heart failure or for ventricular tachyarrhythmias. In fact, the basic questions when and how to treat have also not been resolved for these two conditions.

The symposium "Heart Failure and Arrhythmias" was dedicated to these problems and covered both theoretical topics, such as pathophysiology and pathogenesis, and clinical ones, including prognostic implications.

The symposium was designed as an international satellite workshop to the World Congress of Clinical Pharmacology, which took place in Heidelberg/Mannheim from 23–29 July 1989. It was organized by J. Brachmann and R. Dietz, who were supported by T. Beyer, M. Haass, K.J. Osterziel, A. Pfeifer, C. Schmitt, W. Waas, and B. Waldecker.

The symposium has been made possible by an educational grant from ICI-Pharma, Plankstadt, Federal Republic of Germany. We are very grateful to both the organizers and the sponsors.

Heidelberg, Mai 1990　　　　　　　　　　　　　　　　J. BRACHMANN
　　　　　　　　　　　　　　　　　　　　　　　　　　R. DIETZ
　　　　　　　　　　　　　　　　　　　　　　　　　　W. KÜBLER

Contents

I Pathophysiology

Editorial:
Heart Failure and Arrhythmias
H. Just 3

Pathogenesis of Impaired Pump Function
in Congestive Heart Failure
A.M. Katz (With 1 Figure) 8

Pathogenesis of Ventricular Arrhythmias in Heart Failure
M.J. Janse, J.M.T. de Bakker, and T. Opthof (With 2 Figures) . 16

Evaluation of the Severity of Heart Failure:
Role of Compensatory Mechanisms
R. Dietz, T. Fischer, M. Haass, K.J. Osterziel, and W. Waas
(With 7 Figures) 24

Tissue Renin-Angiotensin Systems in the Pathophysiology
of Heart Failure
A.T. Hirsch and V.J. Dzau (With 1 Figure and 1 Table) 33

Evaluation of the Severity of Ventricular Rhythm
Disturbances: Value of Electrophysiological Testing
and Recording of Late Potentials
L. Seipel, G. Breithardt, and M. Borggrefe
(With 3 Figures and 1 Table) 43

II Approaches to Treatment

Hemodynamic Approach

Editorial:
How to Treat – The Hemodynamic Approach
K. Kochsiek 53

Structural Basis of Left Ventricular Dysfunction:
Role of Collagen Network Remodeling
and Potential Therapeutic Interventions
M.A. SILVER and K.T. WEBER (With 2 Figures)   54

Treatment of Heart Failure by "Afterload" Reduction:
Vasodilator or Angiotensin Converting Enzyme Inhibitor?
P.A. POOLE-WILSON (With 2 Figures and 3 Tables)   66

Possible Role of Positive Inotropic Drugs
in Congestive Heart Failure and in Left Ventricular Dysfunction
H. POULEUR (With 1 Table)   76

Prognostic Indices and Prolongation of Life
K. SWEDBERG (With 2 Figures)   83

Antiarrhythmic Approach

Editorial:
Heart Failure and Malignant Ventricular Arrhythmias
A.J. CAMM   91

Heart Failure and Ventricular Arrhythmias –
The Antiarrhythmic Approach
B. LÜDERITZ (With 1 Figure and 1 Table)   93

When to Treat Arrhythmias in Heart Failure?
A.P.M. GORGELS, P. BRUGADA, and H.J.J. WELLENS
(With 6 Figures and 1 Table) 100

Antiarrhythmic Drugs in Heart Failure
J. BRACHMANN, C. SCHMITT, T. BEYER, B. WALDECKER, T. HILBEL,
M. SCHWEIZER, and W. KÜBLER (With 3 Figures and 2 Tables) . 111

Nonpharmacologic Therapy
for Malignant Ventricular Tachyarrhythmias in Patients
with Congestive Heart Failure
S. SAKSENA (With 4 Figures) 119

Role of Antiarrhythmic Drug Therapy in Patients
with Congestive Heart Failure
R.L. WOOSLEY (With 4 Figures and 3 Tables) 136

III Prognosis

Obtaining Reliable Information
from Randomized Controlled Trials in Congestive Heart Failure
and Left Ventricular Dysfunction
S. Yusuf (With 4 Tables) 147

Prognostic Significance of Asymptomatic Ventricular
Arrhythmias in Heart Failure: Potential for Mortality Reduction
by Pharmacologic Control
B.N. Singh, M.P. Schoenbaum, M. Antimisiaris,
and C. Takanaka (With 3 Figures) 161

Subject Index 175

List of Contributors

ANTIMISIARIS, M., MD
Division of Cardiology 691/111E, VA Medical Center
of West Los Angeles
Wilshire and Sawtelle Boulevards, Los Angeles, CA 90073, USA

BAKKER, J.M.T. DE, MD
Department of Clinical and Experimental Cardiology and the
Interuniversity Cardiology Institute, Academisch Medisch Centrum
Meibergdreef 9, 1105 AZ Amsterdam ZO, The Netherlands

BEYER, T., MD
Department of Internal Medicine III, Medizinische Universitätsklinik
Bergheimer Str. 58, 6900 Heidelberg, FRG

BORGGREFE, M., MD
Department of Internal Medicine C, Medizinische Universitätsklinik
Albert-Schweitzer-Str., 4400 Münster, FRG

BRACHMANN, J., MD
Department of Internal Medicine III, Cardiology
Medizinische Universitätsklinik
Bergheimer Str. 58, 6900 Heidelberg, FRG

BREITHARDT, G., MD
Department of Internal Medicine C, Medizinische Universitätsklinik
Albert-Schweitzer-Str., 4400 Münster, FRG

BRUGADA, P., MD
Department of Cardiology, University Hospital Maastricht
University of Limburg
P.O. Box 1918, 6201 BX Maastricht, The Netherlands

CAMM, A.J., MD
Department of Cardiological Sciences
St. George's Hospital Medical School
London SW17 ORE, UK

DIETZ, R., MD
Department of Internal Medicine III, Cardiology
Medizinische Universitätsklinik
Bergheimer Str. 58, 6900 Heidelberg, FRG

DZAU, V.J., MD
Cellular Vascular Research Laboratory
Brigham and Women's Hospital
Harvard Medical School
75 Francis Street, Boston, MA 02115, USA

FISCHER, T., MD
Department of Internal Medicine III, Medizinische Universitätsklinik
Bergheimer Str. 58, 6900 Heidelberg, FRG

GORGELS, A.P.M., MD
Department of Cardiology, University Hospital Maastricht
University of Limburg
P.O. Box 1918, 6201 BX Maastricht, The Netherlands

HAASS, M., MD
Department of Internal Medicine III, Cardiology
Medizinische Universitätsklinik
Bergheimer Str. 58, 6900 Heidelberg, FRG

HILBEL, T., MD,
Department of Internal Medicine III, Medizinische Universitätsklinik
Bergheimer Str. 58, 6900 Heidelberg, FRG

HIRSCH, A.T., MD
Cardiovascular Physiology Laboratory
Brigham and Women's Hospital
Harvard Medical School
75 Francis Street, Boston, MA 02115, USA

JANSE, M.J., MD
Department of Clinical and Experimental Cardiology and the
Interuniversity Cardiology Institute, Academisch Medisch Centrum
Meibergdreef 9, 1105 AZ Amsterdam ZO, The Netherlands

JUST, H., MD
Department of Internal Medicine III, Cardiology
Hugstetter Str. 55, 7800 Freiburg i. Br., FRG

KATZ, A.M., MD
Cardiology Division, Department of Medicine
University of Connecticut
Farmington, CT 06032, USA

List of Contributors

Kochsiek, K., MD
Department of Internal Medicine, Luitpoldkrankenhaus
Josef-Schneider-Str. 2, 8700 Würzburg, FRG

Kübler, W., MD
Department of Internal Medicine III, Cardiology
Medizinische Universitätsklinik
Bergheimer Str. 58, 6900 Heidelberg, FRG

Lüderitz, B., MD
Department of Internal Medicine, Cardiology
Sigmund-Freud-Str. 25, 5300 Bonn, FRG

Opthof, T., MD
Department of Clinical and Experimental Cardiology and the
Interuniversity Cardiology Institute, Academisch Medisch Centrum
Meibergdreef 9, 1105 AZ Amsterdam ZO, The Netherlands

Osterziel, K.J., MD
Department of Internal Medicine III, Medizinische Universitätsklinik
Bergheimer Str. 58, 6900 Heidelberg, FRG

Poole-Wilson, P.A., MD
Department of Cardiac Medicine, National Heart and Lung Institute
Dovehouse Street, London SW3 6LY, UK

Pouleur, H., MD
Department of Physiology and Division of Cardiology
University of Louvain School of Medicine
Ave. Hippocrate 55 HEDY/5560, 1200 Brussels, Belgium

Saksena, S., MD
Section of Cardiac Electrophysiology, Division of Cardiology
UMDNJ-NJ Medical School, The Eastern Heart Institute
Beth Israel Medical Center
Newark and Passaic, NJ 07055, USA

Schmitt, C., MD
Department of Internal Medicine III, Medizinische Universitätsklinik
Bergheimer Str. 58, 6900 Heidelberg, FRG

Schoenbaum, M.P., MD
Division of Cardiology 691/111E, VA Medical Center
of West Los Angeles
Wilshire and Sawtelle Boulevards, Los Angeles, CA 90073, USA

Schweizer, M., MD
Department of Internal Medicine III, Medizinische Universitätsklinik
Bergheimer Str. 58, 6900 Heidelberg, FRG

SEIPEL, L., MD
Department of Internal Medicine III, Medizinische Universitätsklinik
Auf dem Schnarrenberg, 7400 Tübingen, FRG

SILVER, M.A., MD
Cardiovascular Institute, Michael Reese Hospital
University of Chicago, Pritzker School of Medicine
Chicago, IL 60616, USA

SINGH, B.N., MD
Division of Cardiology 691/111E, VA Medical Center
of West Los Angeles
Wilshire and Sawtelle Boulevards, Los Angeles, CA 90073, USA

SWEDBERG, K., MD
Department of Internal Medicine, Gothenburg University
Östra Hospital, 41685 Gothenburg, Sweden

TAKANAKA, C., MD
Division of Cardiology 691/111E, VA Medical Center
of West Los Angeles
Wilshire and Sawtelle Boulevards, Los Angeles, CA 90073, USA

WAAS, W., MD
Department of Internal Medicine III, Medizinische Universitätsklinik
Bergheimer Str. 58, 6900 Heidelberg, FRG

WALDECKER, B., MD
Department of Internal Medicine III, Medizinische Universitätsklinik
Bergheimer Str. 58, 6900 Heidelberg, FRG

WEBER, K.T., MD
Cardiovascular Institute, Michael Reese Hospital
University of Chicago, Pritzker School of Medicine
Chicago, IL 60616, USA

WELLENS, H.J.J., MD
Department of Cardiology, University Hospital Maastricht
University of Limburg
P.O. Box 1918, 6201 BX Maastricht, The Netherlands

WOOSLEY, R.L., MD
Department of Pharmacology, Georgetown
University School of Medicine, Washington, DC 20007, USA

YUSUF, S., MD
Clinical Trials Branch, Division of Epidemiology
and Clinical Applications, National Heart, Lung and Blood Institute
Bethesda, MD 20892, USA

I Pathophysiology

Editorial:
Heart Failure and Arrhythmias

H. JUST

The failing heart syndrome is characterized by high mortality. Death in chronic heart failure may be due to progressive pump failure, or it may represent arrhythmic, sudden cardiac death (approximately 40%–50% of cases). While progression to irreversible pump failure can in some cases be halted with vasodilator therapy, in particular with ACE inhibitors, the treatment of arrhythmias and the prevention of arrhythmic death continue to pose a formidable problem and a clinical challenge.

Left ventricular hypertrophy and dysfunction are accompanied by a high incidence of ventricular arrhythmias, the frequency and complexity (Lown classification) of which herald the risk of ventricular tachyarrhythmias and fibrillation. The reason for the increased tendency to develop ventricular ectopic activity and for the increased myocardial vulnerability is only incompletely understood, although several factors are well known (see below). The treatment of ventricular arrhythmias in heart failure meets with particular difficulties due to the inherent negative inotropic effect of almost all anti-arrhythmic agents and to a pronounced proarrhythmic effect of these agents especially under the conditions of heart failure.

Left ventricular dysfunction comprises a broad spectrum of myocardial structural and metabolic changes. In addition to local, intramyocardial anatomic and biochemical alterations, one sees changes in central and peripheral hemodynamics (wall tension and stress, pulmonary congestion), hormonal changes with increased sympathetic tone, and changes in electrolyte balance. Therefore, left ventricular dysfunction is related to the genesis of ventricular arrhythmias by many different mechanisms.

It has been shown that increases both in muscle mass and in myocardial fibrosis are related to the genesis of ventricular arrhythmias, and that ventricular arrhythmias originate in areas adjacent to scar or fibrotic tissue. When these areas are examined histologically, viable myocardial cells are seen to be imbedded in scar tissue. It is probable that slow conduction, conduction block, and decremental conduction, as well as heterogeneous spread of the excitation, develop within such areas. These regions lend themselves as the anatomical and electrophysiological substrate for reentrant arrhythmias, frequently for multiple pathway reentrant arrhythmias. It has also been shown that hypoxemia or ischemia are likely to occur in the border zone between viable myocardium and necrotic or scar tissue. Both hypoxemia and ischemia further aggravate electrical instability. Various electrophysiological mechanisms are considered responsible, such as oscillating changes in the resting membrane potential and triggered activity.

There is convincing evidence that hypertrophy in itself alters the electrophysiological properties of the tissue in a way that predisposes to arrhythmias. It has been demonstrated that action potential duration increases significantly in the hypertrophied myocardium. It has likewise been demonstrated that these electrical changes predispose to the development of the late after-depolarizations and triggered activity. Hypertrophy increases not only the propensity for development of arrhythmias but also ventricular fibrillation, i.e., it lowers the ventricular fibrillation threshold. Ventricular fibrillation occurs more frequently if ventricular hypertrophy is present.

In left ventricular dysfunction due to coronary artery disease intermittent ischemia is likely to play a major role in the genesis of ventricular arrhythmias. Numerous studies have shown that ischemia is more frequently associated with arrhythmias if heart failure is present. In this situation, not only electrical changes but also mechanical abnormalities result from reduced blood supply in localized areas of the myocardium. It has been postulated that a common mechanism, the increase in myoplasmic calcium concentration, might be responsible for both the impairment of relaxation and contraction and for the genesis of ventricular arrhythmias. Such an increase in myoplasmic calcium can produce arrhythmias due to delayed conduction as well as to triggered activity. The mechanical alterations of the myocardium may by themselves increase the propensity to develop arrhythmias further, for example, due to increased ventricular wall stress or tension. With progressive left ventricular dysfunction, not only does myocardial tension increase, but a variety of neurohumoral mechanisms are activated. Especially the regularly increased sympathetic tone, due to decreased cardiac output, increased wall tension, and increased pulmonary blood volume (elevated blood pressure in the pulmonary artery!) tend to stimulate heart rate and myocardial contractility. Elevated plasma catecholamine concentrations are assumed to be directly arrhythmogenic. In many different experimental preparations and conditions catecholamines have been shown to increase the magnitude of delayed after-depolarizations, increasing the susceptibility to triggered automaticity. Stimulation of the β_2-receptors by increased endogenous catecholamine levels may induce hypokalemia, a very potent arrhythmia-producing factor. Hypokalemia at the same time lowers the ventricular fibrillation threshold.

Coronary Artery Disease

A number of studies have shown a strong positive correlation between the severity of ventricular arrhythmias and both the extent of coronary artery disease, on the one hand, and the degree of left ventricular dysfunction, on the other. Most of these studies included patients with previous myocardial infarction. It has been shown that the number of scars, extent of single infarcted areas, and occurrence of aneurysms correlate with the incidence and severity of arrhythmias. There is also a correlation with the overall ejection fraction.

Acute Myocardial Infarction

In acute infarction a positive correlation seems to exist between the degree of left ventricular dysfunction and the presence of complex ventricular arrhythmias and the incidence of ventricular fibrillation.

Postmyocardial Infarction

Two multicenter trials have evaluated the relationship between left ventricular dysfunction, ventricular arrhythmias, and mortality after acute myocardial infarction. That of MILIS included 533 postmyocardial infarct patients and the MPIP study included 766 patients. These compared left ventricular ejection fraction as determined by radionuclide angiography and the findings of 24-h Holter monitoring at the time of hospital discharge. According to pooled data from these studies, left ventricular dysfunction and arrhythmias were significantly correlated, however not very strongly so. By univariate analyses of risk factors, repetitive ventricular arrhythmias, and left ventricular ejection fraction below 40%, subsequent mortality could be well predicted. In both studies the relation to mortality was demonstrated after adjusting for left ventricular dysfunction using a cut-off point for ejection fraction at 40%. These correlations, however, were not very strong. Other, individual factors had to be taken into account. Since not all subsets of patients with coronary artery disease carry the same risk of dying suddenly, the question remains as to whether additional factors may be of importance. One such factor may be the appearance of symptomatic or asymptomatic (silent) myocardial ischemia. It has been shown repeatedly that the incidence of ventricular ectopic activity increases with the incidence of symptomatic or asymptomatic ischemic episodes. Furthermore, there is a very strong parallelism in the circadian variation in incidence of ventricular ectopic activity, time of occurrence of sudden cardiac death, onset of acute myocardial infarction, thrombocyte aggregability, fibrinopeptide A levels, and incidence of symptomatic or asymptomatic ischemic episodes.

As regards the coincidence of ventricular dysfunction and ventricular arrhythmias many others have described a significant relationship between the presence of wall motion abnormalities at rest and high-grade ventricular arrhythmias. The best predictor of high-grade arrhythmias is probably a reduced left ventricular ejection fraction, which deteriorates with exercise. In such patients complex arrhythmias under exercise are seen in 60% of the cases, while only 25% of patients with depressed ejection fractions at rest without deterioration under exercise exhibit such arrhythmias.

The mechanisms for the association of exercise-induced depression of left ventricular ejection fraction and increased occurrence of complex arrhythmias are probably related to exercise-induced ischemia, local increases in wall tension, and increased adrenergic tone.

The extraordinary degree of variability of structural changes in the myocardium of patients with coronary artery disease together with the ever-changing pattern of coronary stenosis and dynamic changes in coronary conductance and flow has prevented a more precise picture of predictive factors concerning sudden cardiac death in this disease.

Valvular Heart Disease

In recent years the relationship between ventricular arrhythmias and left ventricular dysfunction has been studied in patients with valve disease using Holter recordings. It could be shown that the occurrence of ventricular arrhythmias was not related to the type of valvular lesion, nor was it related to the transvalvular gradient in aortic stenosis or to the degree of regurgitation. There was, however, a negative correlation between the complexity of ventricular arrhythmias and left ventricular ejection fraction. A positive correlation could also be demonstrated between peak systolic left ventricular wall stress and the incidence of arrhythmias. Similarly, the frequency of ventricular ectopic activity was negatively correlated with the ejection fraction in all types of valve disease.

Our own studies have demonstrated that in 92 patients with aortic and 68 with mitral valve disease the incidence and severity of ventricular arrhythmias were negatively related to left ventricular ejection fraction and positively to left ventricular end-systolic volume index as well as to peak systolic left ventricular wall stress. In aortic regurgitation the frequency of ventricular ectopic beats was negatively correlated to the ejection fraction and positively to the left ventricular end-systolic volume index. These results led us to conclude that the incidence and severity of ventricular arrhythmias in aortic valve disease are determined mainly by the degree of reduction in ejection fraction, increased end-systolic volume index, and augmented peak systolic wall stress. In mitral stenosis no significant correlation between the incidence of ventricular arrhythmias and left ventricular function could be detected. In mitral regurgitation, a significant correlation was found. Here, as in other studies, the ejection fraction was correlated inversely with the incidence and severity of ventricular arrhythmias.

Idiopathic Dilated Cardiomyopathy

In recent years many studies have emerged documenting the correlation between incidence of serious ventricular arrhythmias and the risk of dying suddenly in patients with this disease. Most patients at risk have a severely impaired left ventricular function and exhibit left ventricular hypertrophy.

We have studied 110 consecutive patients with cardiomyopathy according to the Goodwin and Oakley criteria. Upon entrance into the study all patients underwent complete hemodynamic and angiographic study, as well as 24-h monitoring. Of these patients 94% had ventricular arrhythmias, and 45% had episodes of non-sustained ventricular tachycardia. No correlation was found between the severity of clinical heart failure and arrhythmic events. According to the degree of impairment of left ventricular function the patients were divided into three groups: ejection fraction over 50%, between 35% and 50%, and under 35%. A significant inverse correlation could be demonstrated between the ejection fraction and the total number of premature ventricular contractions. During follow-up 39 patients died, 14 from heart failure and 25 suddenly, i.e., of arrhythmias. The deaths occurred 12 ± 7 months after Holter monitoring. The average number of ventricular tachycardia episodes, ventricular pairs, and extrasystoles were compared in survivors and in those who died suddenly or from congestive heart failure; no significant differences were found. The hemodynamic characteristics of the three groups showed that ejection fraction and cardiac index were higher in survivors then in those who died. No differences in any of the variables were found between the patients who died from congestive heart failure as compared to those who died suddenly. These findings suggest that patients with cardiomyopathy and reduced left ventricular ejection fraction (under 35%) and in whom frequent episodes of ventricular tachycardia or ventricular pairs can be detected by 24-h Holter monitoring are at high risk of sudden cardiac death.

Although in all three types of heart disease presented here, a significant correlation between the degree of left ventricular dysfunction and ventricular ectopic activity, on the one hand, and the incidence of arrhythmic cardiac death, on the other, could be demonstrated, prognosis in the individual patient remains difficult. It can be stated, however, that an ejection fraction under 35% in the presence of left ventricular hypertrophy, together with Lown class IVb ventricular arrhythmias or non-sustained ventricular tachycardias characterizes the patient at risk.

The therapeutic consequence of this prognostic definition remains unclear. Beta-blockers would be considered most appropriate, however they are tolerated by only a minority of patients in this group and here only if administered in very small doses. The preventive aspect of this kind of treatment has not been sufficiently investigated. The use of conventional antiarrhythmic agents has not been convincingly demonstrated to be successful as a preventive measure. The CAST study has recently highlighted the dilemma. Only in the case of amiodarone can a preventive effect be considered probable. In 18 cases of repeated occurrence of sustained ventricular tachycardias, after sudden cardiac death with successful resuscitation and in which other antiarrhythmic modalities of treatment had been shown to be unsuccessful, the implantation of an automatically discharging cardioverter/defibrillator had to be considered. This new mode of treatment may provide us with a powerful tool for the treatment of patients at high risk regardless of the underlying etiology of left ventricular dysfunction and ventricular arrhythmia.

Pathogenesis of Impaired Pump Function in Congestive Heart Failure

A. M. Katz

Introduction

The clinical syndrome of congestive heart failure can result from a variety of pathophysiological processes. Overloading of the functioning cells of the failing heart occurs in virtually all of these conditions, most important of which are the dilated and hypertrophic cardiomyopathies, ischemic heart disease, hypertensive heart disease, and valvular heart disease. Chronic overload has at least two important consequences. The first is an increase in the work of the cells of the overloaded myocardium, which increases their energy needs. At the same time that myocardial energy demands are increased in the patient with congestive heart failure, energy production appears to be impaired. Together, these abnormalities can lead to a chronic energy deficit that impairs pump performance in these patients and may contribute to the deterioration and death of the cells of the failing heart.

The cellular hypertrophy that results from chronic overloading is also accompanied by alterations in the structure and function of the hypertrophied myocardium, some of which appear to contribute to the weakness and progressive deterioration of the failing heart. These detrimental consequences of the response to chronic overloading in patients with congestive heart failure can be viewed as a cardiomyopathy of overload that contributes to the downhill course and eventual death of these patients [1].

Is the Failing Heart an Energy-Starved Heart?

It is well established that the number of capillaries supplying the hypertrophied heart does not increase in proportion to the increased mass of muscle [2–3]. The resulting deficit in the availability of substrates needed to generate the chemical energy for contraction and relaxation of the chronically overloaded heart is likely to impair function and hasten cell death in the failing myocardium. More recent electron microscopic studies have confirmed that the number of transverse capillary profiles per square millimeter is decreased in the hypertrophied myocardium [4], which provides further evidence that the failing heart is in an energy-starved state.

Biochemical and morphometric studies of the hypertrophied heart have demonstrated changes in cell composition which also indicate that the hypertrophied heart is in an energy-starved organ [4–8]. Parallel biochemical [7] and morphological [8] studies of the pressure-overloaded rat heart have demonstrated that the fraction of cell volume occupied by energy-consuming myofibrils is increased in the later stages of myocardial hypertrophy, whereas the mass of mitochondria, which generate ATP, is decreased. Thus, both impaired delivery of substrates, notably oxygen, and a disproportionately increased content of contractile proteins relative to mitochondria could contribute to a deficit of chemical energy in the failing heart.

Evidence that the failing human heart is in an anaerobic state is found in the classical studies of Bing [9], which provided evidence that the increased energy demands of the failing human heart are met by increased oxygen extraction rather than increased coronary flow. Decreased myocardial contents of high-energy phosphates have been observed in animal models of heart failure following pressure overloading of the left [10–13] and right [14] ventricles. Endomyocardial biopsies in human hearts have shown a decreased content of high-energy phosphates [15–17] that correlates with the extent to which contraction (inotropy) and relaxation (lusitropy) are impaired [17]. These observations are consistent with the view that an energy deficit contributes to the functional impairment and spontaneous deterioration that occur in the chronically overloaded myocardium.

Functional Consequences of an Energy Deficit in the Failing Heart

While contraction and relaxation are both energy-requiring processes, energy is used quite differently in the systolic and diastolic phases of the cardiac cycle. During systole, the energy needed to power the interactions between the contractile proteins that generate muscular work is derived from ATP, which releases chemical energy when the terminal phosphate bond is hydrolysed by the contractile proteins, myosin and actin. Thus the energy-consuming interactions between actin and myosin allow transduction of the chemical energy of ATP to generate the mechanical energy that allows the heart to propel blood under pressure into the aorta and pulmonary artery. However, energy is also needed for the active transport of Ca^{2+} that allows the heart to relax.

Systole is initiated by the delivery of activator Ca^{2+} to the cytosol of the heart from regions of high Ca^{2+} concentration in the sarcoplasmic reticulum; a smaller entry of Ca^{2+} from the extracellular space contributes to this activator Ca^{2+} but has a more important role in triggering Ca^{2+} release from the sarcoplasmic reticulum. The Ca^{2+} concentration in the cytosol of the resting heart is much lower than in the sarcoplasmic reticulum and extracellular space, the sources of the activator Ca^{2+}; as a result, the initiation of cardiac contraction is mediated by passive, downhill, fluxes of Ca^{2+} down an electrochemical gradient. Conversely, relaxation requires that the heart expend energy to pump the activator Ca^{2+} uphill, out of the cytosol into the sarcoplasmic reticulum and extracellular space [18, 19]. For this reason, although ATP is hydrolyzed by the contractile proteins during contraction, energy is also needed for relaxation of the heart.

The downhill Ca^{2+} fluxes that initiate systole are much more rapid than the active transport processes that cause the heart to relax. Activation involves the extremely rapid processes of diffusion, Ca^{2+} entry via a single sarcolemmal Ca^{2+} channel being approximately 3 000 000 ions per second [20], while the ATP-dependent ion pumps that transport Ca^{2+} uphill, out of the cytosol, are much slower; Ca^{2+} flux through a single sarcoplasmic reticulum Ca^{2+} pump site is approximately 30 ions per second [21], 1/100 000 the rate of Ca^{2+} entry through a Ca^{2+} channel. Even though there are many more Ca^{2+} pump sites than Ca^{2+} channels in the heart, the "reserve" for the Ca^{2+} fluxes involved in relaxation is very much less than for the Ca^{2+} fluxes that activate contraction [22].

Effects of Energy Depletion on Cardiac Function

The complexity of the effects of energy depletion on contraction and relaxation reflect the fact that ATP has two very different effects on cellular systems: substrate effects and allosteric effects.

Substrate Effects of ATP. The most obvious effects of ATP are its substrate effects, where the nucleotide serves as an energy donor. The ATP concentrations needed to saturate the ATPase sites for most energy-consuming reactions are quite low – less than 0.1% of the resting ATP levels in normal myocardium. For this reason, a fall in ATP concentration to levels so low as to deplete substrate ATP probably does not occur in the heart until just before the moment of death. However ATP also exerts important allosteric effects that are seen at much higher ATP concentrations than those which saturate the substrate-binding sites of the proteins that utilize ATP as a source of energy.

Allosteric Effects of ATP. The most important of the allosteric effects of ATP maintain the heart in a state of relaxation. The high ATP concentrations needed to exert these allosteric effects have an important "plasticizing" effect on the contractile proteins by dissociating actin and myosin, thereby maintaining the heart in a relaxed state [23]. Another allosteric effect of high ATP concentrations accelerates turnover of the CA^{2+} pump of the sarcoplasmic reticulum [24, 25]. Attenuation of this effect by a modest fall in ATP levels in the energy-depleted heart would slow the Ca^{2+} pump of the sarcoplasmic reticulum; the resulting slowing of Ca^{2+} transport out of the cytosol would impair relaxation. The Na^+/Ca^{2+} exchanger, which also transports Ca^{2+} out of the cell during diastole, uses the energy of the transsarcolemmal Na^+ gradient, rather than from hydrolysis of ATP, for the active transport of Ca^{2+}. Because the Na^+/Ca^{2+} exchanger is also stimulated by an allosteric effect of high ATP concentrations [26], an energy deficit could slow this ion transport system as well. Thus, even a small decrease in ATP level could impair relaxation because of decreased allosteric effects of ATP to dissociate the contractile proteins, to stimulate the Ca^{2+} pump, and to promote Na^+/Ca^{2+} exchange.

In the failing heart, where an imbalance between energy production and energy utilization is likely to reduce high-energy phosphate levels, the effects on mechanical function would be expected to arise mainly from attenuation of these allosteric effects of ATP. A more severe fall in ATP, to levels where this nucleotide could no longer serve as energy donor for the active transport of Ca^{2+} out of the cytosol, would cause the heart to develop rigor (the "stone heart"), which is the low-energy-state of muscle [27, 28].

Deterioration of the Overloaded Heart

Meerson [29], who first characterized the biochemical events that lead to deterioration and cell death in the overloaded myocardium, described three stages in the response of the heart to a sustained overload. The first, "transient breakdown," is characterized hemodynamically by acute pulmonary congestion and low cardiac output; the heart during this stage exhibits left ventricular dilatation and early hypertrophy. Subsequently, as the ventricle hypertrophies, the increased left ventricular mass alleviates the pulmonary congestion and allows cardiac output to increase, leading to a second stage of "stable hyperfunction." However, the compensation to the chronic overload made possible by hypertrophy does not last, but is followed by progressive left ventricular failure in a third stage that Meerson called "exhaustion and progressive cardiosclerosis." This deterioration of the hypertrophied heart is caused by progressive myocardial fibrosis and cell death that leads ultimately to the death of the animals.

The complex process by which the hypertrophy initiated by overload begins as a compensatory response and then progresses to an inexorable downhill course that ultimately causes the death of the organism can be viewed as a cardiomyopathy of overload (Fig. 1). Seen probably in all patients with chronic congestive heart failure, the cardiomyopathy that accompanies the hypertrophic response to myocardial overloading represents a major cause of progressive disability and death in patients with congestive heart failure [1]. While progressive deterioration

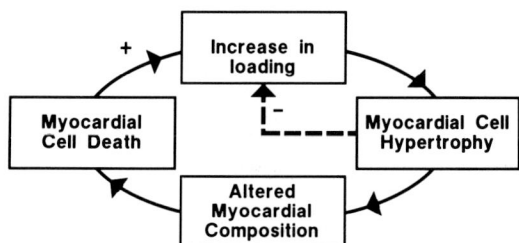

Fig. 1. By increasing the number of contractile units, and so reducing the loading on each sarcomere of the overloaded heart (−), hypertrophy is beneficial. However, hypertrophy also initiates myocardial changes that lead ultimately to cell death. As a result, hypertrophy perpetuates a vicious cycle that, by reducing the number of contractile units, increases the load on each of the surviving cells (+). (Reprinted from [1])

of the hypertrophied heart may be due in part to chronic energy starvation (see above), recent data raise the possibility that molecular changes in the proteins synthesized in the overloaded hearts contribute to this cardiomyopathy.

Abnormal Gene Expression in the Hypertrophied Myocardium

Since Alpert and Gordon [30] first demonstrated that cardiac myosin ATPase activity is depressed in congestive heart failure, a growing number of molecular changes has been documented in the proteins of the hypertrophied heart. At this time, it is not yet known to what extent these alterations in gene expression contribute to, or compensate for, deterioration of the cells of the overloaded heart. Probably, they do both. The appearance of abnormal isoforms of myofibrillar and other myocardial proteins is consistent with the view that the molecular changes caused by altered expression of the genes that encode these proteins contributes to the poor long-term prognosis in patients with congestive heart failure.

Alterations in Myosin. The heavy chains of myosin determine both its ATPase activity (a measure of the rate of energy liberation by myosin in vitro) and muscle shortening velocity (a measure of the rate of energy liberation by myosin in vivo). It is now well established that expression of the genes that encode the cardiac myosin heavy chains is altered by chronic hemodynamic overloading [31–39]. In the rat ventricle, the V1 (α) myosin heavy-chain isoform determines a high myosin ATPase activity and rapid shortening velocity, while the V3 (β) myosin heavy-chain isoform determines a low myosin ATPase activity and slow shortening velocity. In the overloaded heart, preferential synthesis of the V3 myosin heavy chain causes slow myosin to replace fast myosin. Although this alteration in gene expression reduces myocardial contractility by decreasing the rate of cross-bridge cycling [31], it is also accompanied by an increase in mechanical efficiency that exerts an energy-sparing effect [31, 40]. Alterations in myosin gene expression have also been observed in overloaded human hearts [38, 39, 41–44]; and in human atria a decreased proportion of fast (α) atrial myosin heavy chain has been found to parallel the extent of elevation of left atrial pressure [41] and left atrial enlargement [42].

Alterations in other Myocardial Proteins. Synthesis of altered isoforms of actin [45, 46] and tropomyosin [46] has also been found in hypertrophied hearts, where overload leads to the reappearance of isoforms of these proteins that had been predominant during fetal life in the developing heart. The rates at which the altered isoforms of different myofibrillar proteins appear after the heart becomes overloaded demonstrates that the increased protein synthesis that leads to hypertrophy is not simply an up-regulation of sarcomere formation. Instead, the appearance of new myosin and actin isoforms follow different time courses [45, 46], and the newly snythesized protein isoforms appear in different locations. Thus, the newly synthesized β-myosin heavy chains appear first in the inner portions of the left ventricle and around blood vessels, whereas the fetal isoform of actin synthesized in the overloaded heart appears more diffusely throughout the myocardium [47].

Isoform changes in the hypertrophied heart have also been reported for lactate dehydrogenase [48], creatine phosphokinase [49, 50], and the sarcolemmal sodium pump [51]. Reduced calcium uptake by the sarcoplasmic reticulum of the hypertrophied heart, however, appears to reflect a decreased concentration of calcium pump ATPase molecules in this internal membrane rather than expression of an altered isoform of this large molecule [52]. Altered membrane assembly in the hypertrophied heart is also suggested by a recent report that the density of voltage sensitive calcium channels may be increased in the atrial myocardium of patients with hypertrophic cardiomyopathy [53].

Conclusions

Impaired pump function in congestive heart failure can be attributed to at least two quite different mechanisms. The first, an imbalance between energy production and energy utilization in the chronically overloaded cells of the failing heart, can slow many of the processes responsible for ventricular emptying and filling. Energy starvation may also contribute to the deterioration of the overloaded heart that characterizes end-stage congestive heart failure. Abnormal gene expression, which leads to the synthesis of altered cellular constituents in the chronically overloaded heart, also contributes to the negative inotropy and negative lusitropy that impair pump performance in patients with congestive heart failure. In this way, a cardiomyopathy of overload plays a key role in the pathophysiology and clinical course of patients with the diverse clinical syndromes of congestive heart failure.

References

1. Katz AM (1989) Changing strategies in the management of congestive heart failure. J Am Coll Cardiol 13:512–523
2. Shipley RA, Shipley LJ, Wearn JT (1937) The capillary supply in normal and hypertrophied hearts of rabbits. J Exp Med 65:29–42
3. Wearn JT (1939/40) Morphological and functional alterations of the coronary circulation. Harvey Lect 35:243–270
4. Anversa P, Olivetti G, Melissari M, Loud AV (1980) Stereological measurement of cellular and subcellular hypertrophy and hyperplasia in the papillary muscle of adult rat. J Mol Cell Cardiol 12:781–795
5. Wollfenberger A, Schulze W (1962) Über das Volumenverhältnis von Mitochondrien zu Myofibrillen im chronisch überlasteten, hypertrophierten Herzen. Naturwissenschaften 7:161–162
6. Meerson FZ (1961) On the mechanism of compensatory hyperfunction and insufficiency of the heart. Cor Vasa 3:161–177
7. Rabinowitz M (1973) Protein synthesis and turnover in normal and hypertrophied heart. Am J Cardiol 31:202–210

8. Page E, McCalister LP (1973) Quantitative electron microscopic description of heart muscle cells. Application to normal, hypertrophied and thyroxin-stimulated hearts. Am J Cardiol 31:172–181
9. Blain JM, Schafer H, Siegel AL, Bing RJ (1956) Studies on myocardial metabolism. VI. Myocardial metabolism in congestive failure. Am J Med 20:820–833
10. Furchgott RF, Lee KS (1961) High energy phosphates and the force of contraction of cardiac muscle. Circulation 24:416–428
11. Feinstein MB (1962) Effects of experimental congestive heart failure, ouabain, and asphyxia on the high-energy phosphate content of the guinea pig heart. Circ Res 10:333–346
12. Wollenberger A (1962) Losses in mitochondrial mass, structure, and metabolic capacity in the hypertrophied heart prior to failure. Proceedings of the IV World Congress Cardiology, Mexico City, V:275–282
13. Pool PE, Spann JF, Buccino RA, Sonnenblick EH, Braunwald E (1967) Myocardial high energy phosphate stores in cardiac hypertrophy and heart failure. Circ Res 21:365–373
14. Wexler LF, Lorell BH, Monomura S-I, Weinberg EO, Ingwall JS, Apstein CS (1988) Enhanced sensitivity to hypoxia-induced diastolic dysfunction in pressure-overload left ventricular hypertrophy in the rat: role of high-energy phosphate depletion. Circ Res 62:766–775
15. Peyton RB, Jones RN, Attarian D, Sink JD, van Trigt P, Currie WD, Wechsler AS (1982) Depressed high energy phosphate content in hypertrophied ventricles of animal and man. Ann Surg 196:278–283
16. Swain JL, Sabina RL, Peyton RB et al. (1982) Derangements in myocardial purine and pyrimidine nucleotide metabolism in patients with coronary artery disease and left ventricular hypertrophy. Proc Natl Acad Sci USA 79:655–659
17. Bashore TM, Magorien DJ, Letterio J, Shaffer P, Unverferth DV (1987) Histologic and biochemical correlates of left ventricular chamber dynamics in man. J Am Coll Cardiol 9:734–742
18. Tada M, Yamamoto T, Tonomura Y (1978) Molecular mechanisms of active calcium transport by sarcoplasmic reticulum. Physiol Rev 58:1–79
19. Katz AM (1988) Cellular mechanisms in congestive heart failure. Am J Cardiol 62:3A–8A
20. Tsien RW (1983) Calcium channels in excitable cell membranes. Annu Rev Physiol 45:341–358
21. Shigekawa M, Finegan J-AM, Katz AM (1976) Calcium transport ATPase of canine cardiac sarcoplasmic reticulum. A comparison with that of rabbit fast skeletal muscle sarcoplasmic reticulum. J Biol Chem 251:6894–6900
22. Katz AM (1986) Potential deleterious effects of inotropic agents in the therapy of chronic heart failure. Circulation 73 [Suppl III]:III-184–III-188
23. Katz AM (1970) Contractile proteins of the heart. Physiol Rev 50:63–158
24. Shigekawa M, Dougherty JP, Katz AM (1978) Reaction mechanism of Ca^{2+}-dependent ATP hydrolysis by skeletal muscle sarcoplasmic reticulum in the absence of added alkali metal salts. I. Characterization of steady state ATP hydrolysis and comparison with that in the presence of KCl. J Biol Chem 253:1442–1450
25. Nakamura Y, Tonomura Y (1982) The binding of ATP to the catalytic and the regulatory site of Ca^{2+}, Mg^{2+}-dependent ATPase of the sarcoplasmic reticulum. J Bioenerg Biomed 14:307–318
26. DiPolo R (1976) The influence of nucleotides on calcium fluxes. Fed Proc 35:2579–2582
27. Katz AM, Tada M (1972) The "stone heart:" A challenge to the biochemist. Am J Cardiol 29:578–580
28. Katz AM, Tada M (1977) The "stone heart" and other challenges to the biochemist. Am J Cardiol 39:1073–1077
29. Meerson FZ (1961) On the mechanism of compensatory hyperfunction and insufficiency of the heart. Cor Vasa 3:161–177
30. Alpert NR, Gordon MS (1962) Myofibrillar adenosine triphosphatase activity in congestive heart failure. Am J Physiol 202:940–946
31. Hamrell BB, Alpert NA (1986) Cellular basis of the mechanical properties of hypertrophied myocardium. In: Fozzard H, Haber E, Katz A, Jennings R, Morgan HE (eds) The heart and cardiovascular system. Raven, New York, pp 1507–1524
32. Bugaisky L, Zak R (1986) Biological mechanisms of hypertrophy. In: Fozzard H, Haber E, Katz A, Jennings R, Morgan HE (eds) The heart and cardiovascular system. Raven, New York, pp 1491–1506

33. Swynghedauw B (1986) Developmental and functional adaptation of contractile proteins in cardiac and skeletal muscles. Physiol Rev 66:710–771
34. Lompre AM, Schwartz K, D'Albis A, Lacombe G, Van Thiem N, Swynghedauw B (1979) Myosin isoenzyme redistribution in chronic heart overload. Nature 282:105–107
35. Rupp H (1981) The adaptive changes in the isoenzyme pattern of myosin from hypertrophied rat myocardium as a result of pressure overload and physical training. Basic Res Cardiol 76:79–88
36. Scheuer J, Malhotra A, Hirsch C, Capasso J, Schaible TF (1982) Physiologic cardiac hypertrophy corrects contractile protein abnormalities associated with pathologic hypertrophy in rats. J Clin Invest 70:1300–1305
37. Litten RZ, Martin BJ, Low RB, Alpert NR (1982) Altered myosin isozyme pattern from pressure-overloaded and thyrotoxic hypertrophied rabbit hearts. Circ Res 50:856–864
38. Tsuchimochi H, Kuro-o M, Takaku F, Yoshida K, Kawana M, Kimata S-I, Yazaki Y (1986) Expression of myosin isozymes during the developmental stage and their redistribution induced by pressure overload. Jpn Circ J 50:1044–1052
39. Izumo S, Lompre A-M, Matsuoka R, Koren G, Schwartz K, Nadal-Ginard B, Mahdavi V (1987) Myosin heavy chain messenger RNA and protein isoform transitions during cardiac hypertrophy. J Clin Invest 79:970–977
40. Katz AM (1973) Biochemical "defect" in the hypertrophied and failing heart. Deleterious or compensatory? Circulation 47:1076–1079
41. Tschuchimochi H, Sugi M, Kuro-o M, Ueda S, Takaku F, Furuta S-I, Shirai T, Yazaki Y (1984) Isozymic changes in myosin of human atrial myocardium induced by overload. Immunohistochemical study using monoclonal antibodies. J Clin Invest 74:662–665
42. Mercadier JJ, De La Bastie D, Menasche P, N'Guyen Van Cao A, Bouvenet P, Lorente P, Piwnica A, Slama R, Schwartz K (1987) Alpha-myosin heavy chain isoform and atrial size in patients with various types of mitral valve dysfunction: a quantitative study. J Am Coll Cardiol 9:1024–1030
43. Cummins P (1982) Transition in human atrial and ventricular myosin light-chain isozymes in response to cardiac-pressure-overload-induced hypertrophy. Biochem J 205:195–204
44. Kurabayashi M, Komuro I, Tsuchimochi H, Takaku F, Yazaki Y (1988) Molecular cloning and characterization of human atrial and ventricular myosin alkali light chain cDNA clones. J Biol Chem 263:13930–13936
45. Schwartz K, De la Bastie D, Bouveret P, Olivieo P, Alonso S, Buckingham M (1986) α-Skeletal muscle actin mRNA's accumulate in hypertrophied adult rat hearts. Circ Res 59:551–555
46. Izumo S, Nadal-Ginard B, Mahdave V (1988) Protooncogene induction and reprogramming of cardiac gene expression produced by pressure overload. Proc Natl Acad Sci USA 85:339–343
47. Schiaffino S, Samuel JL, Sassoon D, Lompre AM, Garner I, Marotte F, Buckingham M, Rappaport L, Schwartz K (1989) Nonsynchronous accumulation of α-skeletal actin and β-myosin heavy chain mRNAs during early stages of pressure-overloaded-induced cardiac hypertrophy demonstrated by in situ hybridization. Circ Res 64:937–948
48. Fox AC (1971) High-energy phosphate compounds and LDH isozymes in the hypertrophied right ventricle. In: Alpert NR (ed) Cardiac hypertrophy. Academic Press, New York, pp 203–212
49. Meerson FZ, Javick MP (1982) Isozyme pattern and activity of myocardial creatine phosphokinase under heart adaptation to chronic overload. Basic Res Cardiol 77:349–358
50. Ingwall JS, Kramer MF, Fifer MA, Lorell BH, Shemin R, Grossman W, Allen PD (1985) The creatine kinase system in normal and diseased human myocardium. N Engl J Med 313:1050–1054
51. Charlemagne D, Maixen J-M, Preteseille M, Lelievre LG (1986) Ouabain binding sites and (Na^+, K^+)-ATPase activity in rat cardiac hypertrophy: expression of neonatal forms. J Biol Chem 261:185–189
52. Lompre AM, Levitsky D, de la Bastie D, Mercadier J-J, Rappaport L, Schwartz K (1988) Function of the sarcoplasmic reticulum and expression of its Ca^{2+} ATPase gene in pressure overloaded rat myocardium. Circulation 78 [Suppl II]:II-535 (abstr)
53. Wagner JA, Sax FL, Weisman HF, Porterfield J, McIntosh C, Weisfeldt ML, Snyder SH, Epstein SE (1989) Calcium-antagonist receptors in the atrial tissue of patients with hypertrophic cardiomyopathy. N Engl J Med 320:755–761

Pathogenesis of Ventricular Arrhythmias in Heart Failure

M.J. Janse, J.M.T. de Bakker, and T. Opthof

Introduction

There is a large body of clinical evidence that impaired left ventricular function is an important and independent factor identifying the patient with coronary artery disease who is at high risk for sudden cardiac death [1–6]. However, even in the absence of coronary artery disease, heart failure appears to be arrhythmogenic. Patients with congestive heart failure, regardless of etiology, have a high incidence of sudden death and a high incidence of complex arrhythmias [7–14]. Between 30% and 50% of all deaths are sudden, presumably caused by ventricular fibrillation. In some reports the incidence of multiform ventricular premature beats, pairs, or nonsustained ventricular tachycardia is almost 90%. There is now general agreement that in patients with heart failure both the degree of left ventricular dysfunction and the presence of complex ventricular arrhythmias are independent risk factors for mortality [7, 10, 12]. Whereas clinically the relationship between heart failure and arrhythmias is well established, the reasons why this is so are largely unknown. In this chapter we discuss possible arrhythmogenic factors associated with heart failure, bearing in mind that almost certainly there is no single arrhythmogenic factor, and that it is impossible to state precisely in which way the many factors that could cause an arrhythmia interact.

Arrhythmogenic Factors in Heart Failure

Four different categories of arrhythmogenic factors can be considered: (a) neurohumoral factors, particularly increased levels of catecholamines and enhanced activity of the sympathetic nervous system; (b) electrolyte disturbances such as low serum levels for K^+ and Mg^{2+}; (c) medication with antiarrhythmic drugs, cardiac glycosides, diuretics, or inotropic drugs; and (d) mechanical and anatomical factors such as stretch, abnormal wall motion, and myocardial infarction.

There is evidence for increased sympathetic outflow and reduced parasympathetic activity in patients with heart failure [15–17], and the presence of increased levels of circulating catecholamines is associated with a poor prognosis [18]. Enhanced sympathetic activity may lead to hypokalemia, both by uptake of potassium in skeletal muscle [19, 20] and by myocardium [21]. In patients with heart failure low concentrations of potassium were indeed associated with increased plasma levels of catecholamines [8].

The proarrhythmogenic effects of antiarrhythmic drugs, especially of drugs of class Ic [14, 22] are probably related to slowing of conduction, which may predispose to reentrant arrhythmias. The results of studies on the effects of antiarrhythmogenic drug therapy in patients with congestive heart failure are inconclusive, one study showing no effect at all [23], the other a slight reduction in the incidence of arrhythmias [24]. The number of patients studied, however, is too small to draw definite conclusions.

Other forms of therapy may also exacerbate arrhythmias. Diuretics may cause hypokalemia; cardiac glycosides may cause triggered activity (see below); inotropic therapy designed to increase intracellular levels of cyclic AMP, either by promoting synthesis (beta-adrenergic agonists) or by retarding its degradation (phosphodiesterase inhibitors) may cause hypokalemia and increased cytosolic calcium concentration which can cause triggered activity based on delayed afterdepolarization.

The possible arrhythmogenic effects of wall motion abnormalities, stretch, and the anatomical changes caused by infarction are discussed in the following section.

Arrhythmia Substrates

Substrates for Reentry

Generally speaking, ventricular fibrillation is the result of the interaction of a trigger and a substrate, whereas several modulating factors may influence both trigger and substrate. The most likely substrate for ventricular tachycardia or fibrillation is one, or multiple, pathway(s) for reentrant excitation. Evidence obtained from isolated, revived, Langendorff-perfused hearts of patients with extensive myocardial infarction and intractable congestive heart failure who underwent cardiac transplantation indicates that isolated bundles of surviving myocardial cells within the infarct serve as the critical part of a reentrant circuit [25]. When an appropriate trigger is present, for example, a spontaneous or electrically induced premature beat, a reentrant ventricular tachycardia, which eventually may degenerate into fibrillation, occurs.

Figure 1 is a schematic representation of the endocardial surface of the left ventricle of an isolated perfused human heart, where the ventricle is "folded out." The shaded areas indicate zones of healed infarction. In this heart a sustained monomorphic ventricular tachycardia was induced by application of a premature electrical stimulus to the ventricles. The pathway of excitation during one tachycardia cycle is indicated by isochronic lines. Numbers are in milliseconds, relative to an arbitrarily chosen time zero. Cycle length of the tachycardia was 320 ms, and throughout this interval electrical activity was recorded along the pathway indicated by arrows, strongly suggesting that the mechanism of this tachycardia was circus-movement reentry. A critical part of the reentrant circuit was located between the 40- and 60-ms isochrone, in the area where the anterior wall joined the septum. In Fig. 2 schematic drawings are shown of histological sections taken

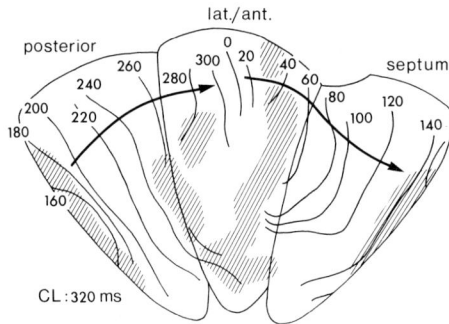

Fig. 1. Activation pattern during a sustained monomorphic ventricular tachycardia in an isolated Langendorff-perfused heart of a patient with coronary heart disease and congestive heart failure who underwent cardiac transplantation. The endocardial surface of the left ventricle is schematically depicted with the heart folded out via an imaginary cut along the posterior descending coronary artery. *Shaded areas*, zones of healed infarction; isochronic lines are drawn at 20-ms intervals; *arrow,* spread of activation during tachycardia, which had a cycle length of 320 ms

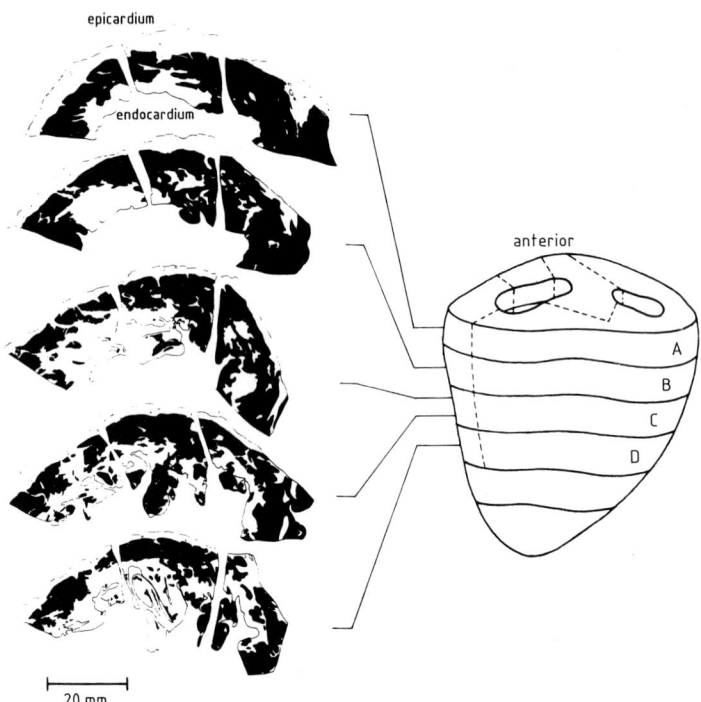

Fig. 2. Schematic drawing of histological sections taken from the area between the 20- and 60-ms isochrone of Fig. 1. Surviving myocardium is indicated in *black,* fibrous tissue in *white.* Only in level A is there a continuous strand of surviving myocardium within the infarct connecting the noninfarcted myocardium to septum and anterior wall. In all other levels connective tissue interrupts bundles of surviving muscle

from base to apex in this area. At each level three separate adjoining sections are shown. Surviving myocardium is shown in black, fibrous tissue in white. Only in the upper level (A) is there continuity of surviving myocardium from right to left. In all other levels (left sections) the bundles of myocardium are separated from each other by fibrous tissue extending from endocardium to epicardium.

Other substrates for reentry may be formed by intermingling of muscle fibers and collagen bundles in hypertrophied hearts, especially in the subendocardium. Since many patients with congestive heart failure who die suddenly showed signs of ischemia in their last week of life [7], and particularly in hypertrophied hearts subendocardial ischemia can occur in response to exertion [26], acutely ischemic myocardium may also provide the substrate for reentry. In dogs coronary artery occlusion in hypertrophied hearts causes ventricular fibrillation more often than in normal hearts, most likely because of an increased size of the ischemic area [27, 28].

The electrophysiological alterations caused by acute ischemia are complex [29], but the main effects responsible for the genesis of reentrant arrhythmias are (a) slowing of conduction, (b) changes in refractory period, and (c) inhomogeneity.

In general, recovery of excitability in the central ischemic zone, where cells are partially depolarized, is prolonged. Cells close to the border with nonischemic myocardium with unchanged or minimally depolarized resting membrane potentials may have refractory periods that are shorter than those of normal myocardium. This results in an increased dispersion of refractoriness within the ischemic area, which is one of the most important reasons for the occurrence of reentry. Increases in heart rate or premature impulses may unmask the electrical inhomogeneity: cells with the longest recovery times show alternation or even block, whereas cells with the shorter refractory periods are still able to respond in a 1:1 fashion. Thus, areas of unidirectional block may be created by a mere increase in heart rate, and the stage may be set for reentry.

Substrates for Focal Activity

Another possibility for an arrhythmia substrate is a focus, that is a group of cells displaying repetitive activity. Focal repetitive activity may be caused by abnormal automaticity or by triggered activity based on either early or delayed afterpotentials. Whereas certain types of focal activity may cause sustained ventricular tachycardia, they may also serve as a trigger for reentrant arrhythmias; we discuss these mechanisms therefore in the next section.

Triggers for Reentry

Triggers for sustained reentry are single or multiple premature impulses or sudden increases in heart rate. There are many ways in which factors associated with heart failure can induce ectopic impulse formation.

Mechanical Factors

The possibility that wall motion abnormalities may influence electrophysiological parameters has been explored by Lab and colleagues [30–34]. In isolated muscle preparations the duration of the intracellular calcium transient was increased when the muscle shortened isotonically. This led to a lengthening of the action potential and in the development of an early afterdepolarization. In regional ischemia the ischemic segment shows out-of-phase movement with lengthening of the ischemic segment during early systole followed by late (isotonic) shortening. Recordings of monophasic potentials showed action potential lengthening and early afterdepolarization which sometimes resulted in a triggered premature impulse.

Other investigators showed that stretch can induce rapid automatic firing in Purkinje fibers and muscle fibers [35, 36]. In healthy subjects ventricular premature beats were found in individuals in whom echocardiography revealed the presence of thick, longitudinal false tendons which supposedly were subjected to mechanical stretch [37].

Adrenergic Simulation and Low Extracellular K^+

The combination of high levels of circulating catecholamines and low levels of potassium may lead to the following electrophysiological alteration. First, the slope of phase 4 depolarization may be enhanced, or automatic activity can be initiated in latent pacemakers [38]. Secondly, both early and delayed afterdepolarizations may occur, each of which can induce single triggered ectopic impulses or a series of repetitive beats [39, 40]. The occurrence of triggered activity based on delayed afterdepolarization becomes even more likely in the presence of digitalis [39]. Low levels of Mg^{2+} may potentiate the arrhythmogenic effects of digitalis [41].

In summary, in patients with congestive heart failure several factors may be present that predispose to enhanced automaticity and triggered activity: abnormal wall motion and mechanical stretch of Purkinje or muscle fibers, adrenergic stimulation, low levels of K^+ and Mg^{2+}, and digitalis.

The electrophysiological effects of these factors have been studied in isolated preparations from hearts that were normal. There are some animal studies, however, indicating that heart failure may induce electrophysiological changes.

Animal Studies on the Electrophysiological Effects of Heart Failure

A number of animal models have been developed to study the electrophysiological consequences of heart failure. Usually, pressure-overloaded ventricles have been produced by obstructing right or left ventricular outflow by banding of either the pulmonary artery or the aorta. Although abnormalities in transmembrane potentials have been found, it is not easy to link these in a straightforward way to arrhythmia mechanisms. Both in hypertrophied cat and rat hearts marked prolongation of the action potential has been measured, with slight but insignificant changes in other parameters [42, 43]. If anything, one would expect a prolongation of the action potential to be antiarrhythmic, at any rate for reentrant arrhythmias. In hypertrophied rat myocardium delayed and early afterdepolarizations and triggered activity have been observed, although the isolated preparations had to be superfused with solutions containing either elevated calcium concentrations or tetraethylammonium [44]. It is not always clear whether the reported changes are primarily characteristic of hypertrophy, and may be unrelated to cardiac failure. There is one report in which a clear distinction is made between hypertrophy with and without heart failure [45]. In hypertrophied hearts of cats with clinical signs of heart failure, resting membrane potential, action potential amplitude and maximum upstroke velocity were markedly reduced. These changes were not found in ventricular muscle of cats with hypertrophy uncomplicated by failure. Another study on hypertrophied left ventricles of cats reported on the presence of fibrotic areas on the endocardial surface with intermingling of viable muscle cells and connective tissue. In these areas relative normal action potentials were interspersed with electrically silent zones and potentials of abnormal configuration: short duration, low amplitude, notched upstrokes, and reduced membrane potentials [46]. The findings of these last two studies point to slow conduction and dispersion of refractoriness, factors predisposing to reentry.

References

1. Cobb LA, Werner JA, Trobaugh GB (1980) Sudden cardiac death. I. A decade's experience with out-of-hospital resuscitation. Mod Concepts Cardiovasc Dis 49:31–36
2. Goldstein S, Landis JR, Leighton R, Ritter G, Vasu CM, Lantis A, Serokman R (1981) Characteristics of the resuscitated out-of-hospital cardiac arrest victim with coronary heart disease. Circulation 64:977–984
3. Myerburg RJ, Conde CA, Sung RJ, Mayorga-Cortes A, Mallon S, Sheps DS, Appel RA, Castellanos A (1980) Clinical, electrophysiologic and hemodynamic profile of patients resuscitated from prehospital cardiac arrest. Am J Med 68:568–576
4. Pitt B (1982) Sudden cardiac death: role of left ventricular dysfunction. Ann NY Acad Sci 382:218–228
5. Schulze RA, Strauss HW, Pitt B (1977) Sudden death in the year following myocardial infarction. Relation to ventricular premature contractions in the late hospital phase and left ventricular function. Am J Med 62:192–199
6. Weaver WD, Lorch GS, Alvarez HA, Cobb LA (1976) Angiographic findings and prognostic indicators in patients resuscitated from sudden cardiac death. Circulation 54:895–900
7. Bigger JT Jr (1987) Why patients with congestive heart failure die: arrhythmias and sudden cardiac death. Circulation 75 [Suppl IV]:28–35
8. Dargie HJ, Cleland JGF, Leckie BJ, Inglis CG, East BW, Ford I (1987) Relation of arrhythmias and electrolyte abnormalities to survival in patients with severe chronic heart failure. Circulation 75 [Suppl IV]:98–107
9. Franciosa JA, Wilen M, Ziesche S, Cohn JN (1983) Survival in men with severe chronic left ventricular failure due to either coronary heart disease or idiopathic dilated cardiomyopathy. Am J Cardiol 51:831–836

10. Holmes J, Kubo SH, Cody RJ, Kligfield P (1985) Arrhythmias in ischemic and non-ischemic dilated cardiomyopathy: prediction of mortality by ambulatory electrocardiomyopathy. Am J Cardiol 55:146–151
11. Lee WH, Packer M (1986) Prognostic importance of serum sodium concentration and its modification by converting-enzyme inhibition in patients with severe chronic heart failure. Circulation 73:257–267
12. Meinertz T, Hoffman T, Kasper W, Treese N, Bechthold H, Stienen U, Pop T, Leitner ERV, Andersen D, Meyer J (1984) Significance of ventricular arrhythmias in idiopathic dilated cardiomyopathy. Am J Cardiol 53:902–907
13. Packer M (1985) Sudden unexpected death in patients with congestive heart failure: a second frontier. Circulation 72:681–685
14. Wilson JR (1987) Use of antiarrhythmic drugs in patients with heart failure: clinical efficacy, hemodynamic results and relation to survival. Circulation 75 [Suppl IV]:64–73
15. Eckberg DL, Drabinsky M, Braunwald E (1971) Defective cardiac parasympathetic control in patients with heart disease. N Engl J Med 285:877–883
16. Saul JP, Arai Y, Berger RD, Lilly LS, Colucci WS, Cohen RJ (1988) Assessment of autonomic regulation in chronic congestive heart failure by heart rate spectral analysis. Am J Cardiol 61:1292–1299
17. Leimbach WN, Wallin BG, Victor RG, Aylward PE, Sundloef G, Mark AL (1986) Direct evidence from intraneural recordings for increased central sympathetic outflow in patients with heart failure. Circulation 73:913–919
18. Cohn JN, Levine TB, Olivari MT, Garberg V, Lura D, Francis GS, Simon AB, Rector T (1984) Plasma norepinephrine as a guide to prognosis in patients with chronic congestive heart failure. N Engl J Med 311:819–823
19. Clausen T (1983) Adrenergic control of Na^+-K^+ homeostasis. Acta Med Scand Suppl 672:111–115
20. Brown MJ, Brown DC, Murphy MB (1983) Hypokalemia from beta 2 receptor stimulation by circulating epinephrine. N Engl J Med 309:1414–1419
21. Ellingsen O, Sejersted OM, Leraand S, Ilebekk A (1987) Catecholamine-induced myocardial potassium uptake mediated by beta 1-adrenoceptors and adenylcyclase activation in the pig. Circ Res 60:540–550
22. Morganroth J, Horowitz LN (1988) Antiarrhythmic drug therapy 1988: for whom, how and where? Am J Cardiol 62:461–465
23. Chakko CS, Gheorghiade M (1985) Ventricular arrhythmias in severe heart failure: incidence, significance, and effectiveness of anti-arrhythmic therapy. Am Heart J 109:497–504
24. Parmley WW, Chatterjee K (1986) Congestive heart failure and arrhythmias: an overview. Am J Cardiol 57:34B–37B
25. De Bakker JMT, Van Capelle FJL, Janse ML, Wilde AAM, Coronel R, Becker AE, Dingemans KP, Van Hemel NM, Hauer RNW (1988) Reentry as a cause of ventricular tachycardia in patients with chronic ischemic heart disease: electrophysiologic and anatomic correlation. Circulation 77:589–606
26. Vatner S (1988) Reduced subendocardial myocardial perfusion as one mechanism for congestive heart failure. Am J Cardiol 62:94E–98E
27. Koyanagi S, Eastham C, Marcus ML (1982) Effects of chronic hypertension and left ventricular hypertrophy on the incidence of sudden cardiac death after coronary artery occlusion in conscious dogs. Circulation 65:1192–1197
28. Koyanagi S, Eastham CL, Harrison PG, Marcus ML (1982) Increased size of myocardial infarction in dogs with chronic hypertension and left ventricular hypertrophy. Circ Res 50:55–62
29. Janse MJ, Wit AL (1989) The electrophysiological mechanisms of ventricular arrhythmias resulting from myocardial ischemia and infarction. Physiol Rev 69:1049–1169
30. Lab MJ (1978) Mechanically dependent changes in action potentials recorded from the intact frog heart. Circ Res 42:519–528
31. Covell JW, Lab MJ, Pavelec R (1981) Mechanical induction of paired action potentials in intact heart in situ. J Physiol (Lond) 320:34P
32. Lab MJ (1982) Stress-strain-related depolarization in the myocardium and arrhythmogenesis in early ischemia. In: Parratt JR (ed) Early arrhythmias resulting from myocardial ischemia. Macmillan, London, pp 81–91

33. Lab MJ, Allen DG, Orchard Ch (1984) The effect of shortening on myoplasmic calcium concentration and on the action potential in mammalian ventricular muscle. Circ Res 55:825–829
34. Lab MJ (1987) Mechano-electric coupling in a myocardium and its possible role in ischaemic arrhythmia. In: Sideman A, Begar R (eds) Activation, metabolism and perfusion of the heart. Nijhoff, Boston, pp 227–239
35. Dudel J, Trautwein W (1954) Das Aktionspotential und Mechanogramm des Herzmuskels unter dem Einfluss der Dehnung. Cardiologia 25:344–362
36. Kaufmann R, Theophile U (1967) Automatie-fördernde Dehnungseffekte an Purkinje-Fäden, Papillarmuskeln und Vorhoftrabekeln von Rhesus-Affen. Pfluegers Arch 291:174–189
37. Suwa M, Hirota Y, Kaku K, Yoneda Y, Nakayama A, Kawamura K, Doi K (1988) Prevalence of the coexistence of left ventricular false tendons and premature ventricular complexes in apparently healthy subjects: a prospective study in the general population. J Am Coll Cardiol 12:910–914
38. Vassalle M (1965) Cardiac pacemaker potentials at different extra- and intracellular K concentrations. Am J Physiol 208:770–775
39. Wit AL, Rosen MR (1986) Afterdepolarization and triggered activity. In: Fozzard HA et al. (eds) The heart and cardiovascular system. Raven, New York, pp 1449–1490
40. Eisner DA, Lederer WJ (1979) Inotropic and arrhythmogenic effects of potassium-depleted solutions on mammalian cardiac muscle. J Physiol 294:255–277
41. Fisch C (1973) Relation of electrolyte disturbances to cardiac arrhythmias. Circulation 47:408–419
42. Guelch RW (1988) The effect of elevated chronic loading on the action potentials of mammalian myocardium. J Mol Cell Cardiol 20:415–520
43. Tritthart H, Luedeke H, Bayer R, Stierle H, Kaufmann R (1975) Right ventricular hypertrophy in the cat – an electrophysiological and anatomical study. J Mol Cell Cardiol 7:163–174
44. Aronson RS (1981) Afterpotentials and triggered activity in hypertrophied myocardium from rats with renal hypertension. Circ Res 48:720–727
45. Gelband H, Bassett AL (1973) Depressed transmembrane potentials during experimentally induced ventricular failure in cats. Circ Res 33:625–634
46. Cameron JS, Myerburg R, Wong SS, Gaide MS, Epstein K, Alvarez R, Gelband H, Guse PA, Bassett AL (1983) Electrophysiological consequences of chronic experimentally induced left ventricular pressure overload. J Am Coll Cardiol 2:481–487

Evaluation of the Severity of Heart Failure: Role of Compensatory Mechanisms

R. Dietz, T. Fischer, M. Haass, K.J. Osterziel, and W. Waas

Introduction

The severity of heart failure is in general expressed either by a grading system or by indices of left ventricular function. However, the correlations between currently used classification systems of heart failure and prognosis are poor, and more important, this stratification does not provide a basis for individually adjusted therapy. Treatment of the cause of heart failure is possible, for example, in cases of valvular heart disease. It is not possible when myocardial pump failure is present – except by complete exchange of the diseased heart.

Thus, our main therapeutic aim is to prevent further haemodynamic deterioration. This can be achieved by detecting and treating mechanisms in heart failure that aggravate and accelerate the impairment of pump function. Specifically, in heart failure there are several vicious circles that contribute to a rapid progression of the disease and hence to a reduction in the length and quality of life. They may also provide targets for therapeutic interventions.

Detrimental Consequences of Increased Ventricular Wall Stress in Heart Failure

The first vicious circle results from an increase in ventricular wall stress, which leads to a decrease in coronary flow, an increase in wall thickness, and an increase of ventricular size (Fig. 1). Each of the three induced changes itself contributes to a further progression of heart failure. Therapeutic interventions, therefore, are directed against these alterations, that is to the:

Prevention of further ventricular enlargement
Prevention of further increases in wall thickness due to progressive interstitial fibrosis and hypertrophy of myocytes
Restoration of impaired coronary flow

In a small pilot study the efficacy of acute afterload reduction on filling pressures and coronary flow was evaluated in a total of nine patients with heart failure (NYHA III–IV), seven with dilative cardiomyopathy, two with ischaemic cardiomyopathy. We investigated the immediate response to afterload reduction induced by enalaprilate (2 mg) administered intravenously.

Evaluation of the Severity of Heart Failure: Role of Compensatory Mechanisms

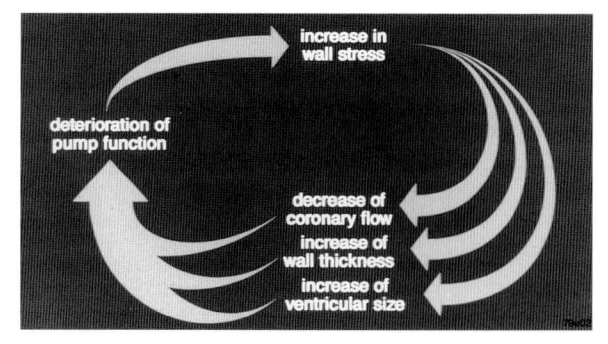

Fig. 1. This vicious circle originates from an increase in wall stress, promoting impairment of coronary flow, enhancement of wall thickness, and enlargement of ventricular size. Each of the three induced changes itself contributes to a further progression of heart failure

Acute angiotensin-converting enzyme (ACE) inhibition in these patients resulted in a fall in right and left ventricular filling pressure by about 30% at rest as well as during physical exercise (50 W in supine position for 2 min). Parameters measuring right and left ventricular filling were improved and cardiac output increased; in addition, coronary flow increased more than 30% both at rest and during physical exercise. This improvement in coronary perfusion in severe heart failure occurred in the presence of reduced energy demand since heart rate was unchanged and blood pressure fell.

Thus, current therapeutic regimens make it possible to ameliorate the otherwise detrimental consequences of the first vicious circle in heart failure by:

1. Reducing wall stress and hence retarding further ventricular enlargement. This effect has been demonstrated in patients suffering from myocardial infarction and treated for 1 year with ACE-inhibitors (compared to controls).
2. Improving impaired coronary perfusion in severe heart failure. This component may be particularly important in patients with ischaemic cardiomyopathy [3–6].
3. Modulating the growth of myocytes and fibroblasts in the failing myocardium. This aspect will be discussed in more detail later in this chapter.

Detrimental Consequences of Stimulated Vasopressor Systems in Heart Failure

A second vicious circle in heart failure is evoked by the stimulation of systems with vasopressor effects (Fig. 2). Although it is believed that stimulated sympathetic activity supports the failing heart and that high angiotensin II and vasopressin levels help to maintain blood pressure, the detrimental effects of these stimulated systems in congestive heart failure (CHF) prevail [7]. An aim of our study therefore was to evaluate the contribution of sympathetic activity to the acute haemodynamic status of patients with different severities of heart failure [8].

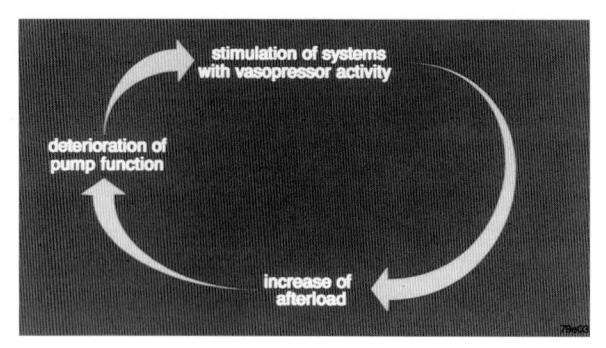

Fig. 2. This vicious circle is evoked by stimulation of vasopressor systems in heart failure. They contribute to the inappropriately elevated systemic vascular resistance. Further deterioration of pump function is the result of the rise in afterload

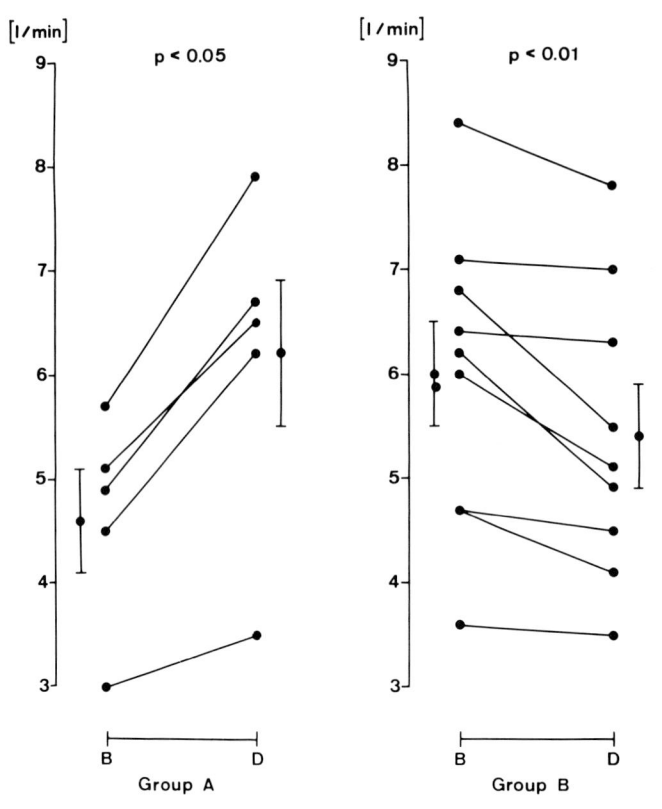

Fig. 3. The response of cardiac output to sudden sympathetic withdrawal by stimulation of baroreceptors is shown for patients with moderate (*Group B*) or severe (*Group A*) heart failure. Whereas cardiac output did not change significantly following baroreceptor stimulation in patients with moderate heart failure, a marked improvement of cardiac output was observed in severe heart failure in response to withdrawal of sympathetic activity

In order to prevent the interaction of drugs with several systems, a non-pharmacological modulation of sympathetic activity was chosen. One way to induce a sudden non-pharmacological withdrawal of sympathetic activity consists of neck suction. By this manoeuvre arterial baroreceptors are stimulated, causing central sympathetic discharge to decrease instantaneously [9, 10].

There was a characteristic time-related response to neck suction. The stimulation of vagal activity occurred immediately and resulted in an increase in the length of the R-R interval. After a 20-s delay the withdrawal of sympathetic activity reached its maximum, as could be seen from the fall in blood pressure. Haemodynamic measurements were then performed.

If an elevated sympathetic tone represented a beneficial mechanism for the failing heart, a sudden further compromise of the haemodynamic status might have been expected when the sympathetic drive was withdrawn acutely. In contrast, if the detrimental effects of sympathetic overactivity outweighed its positive inotropic support, an improvement in cardiac efficacy would occur. Patients with CHF were allocated to one of two groups:

Group A consisted of those with more severe heart failure and elevated plasma noradrenaline levels
Group B consisted of those with moderate heart failure and normal plasma noradrenaline values.

Heart rate responses were qualitatively similar in both groups. Basal heart rates were higher in patients with severe heart failure and increased noradrenaline levels, but these patients exhibited the same fall in heart rate in response to neck suction as did patients with moderate heart failure.

The responses in cardiac output in the two groups were quite different. Whereas a small reduction in cardiac output was observed in patients with moderate heart failure, cardiac output increased by more than 30% in all patients with severe heart failure. This difference was not the consequence of different heart rate responses but was also evident when changes in stroke volume were considered. Sympathetic withdrawal did not change stroke volume in patients with moderate heart failure but significantly improved stroke volume in patients with severe heart failure.

Hence, one may conclude that sympathetic overactivity in patients with severe heart failure contributes to further haemodynamic deterioration. In patients with moderate heart failure, however, the positive inotropic and chronotropic support of the sympathetic system seems to provide a small contribution towards maintaining cardiac output, mainly by accelerating the heart rate.

Sympathetic withdrawal by neck suction can be used for diagnostic purposes but for therapeutic intervention other measures should be utilized. An accepted strategy in heart failure consists of unloading the failing heart. With respect to modulation of sympathetic activity great differences exist between various vasodilator drugs. For example, whereas hydralazine causes sympathetic activity to increase further, sympathetic overactivity is suppressed by ACE inhibition. Suppression of sympathetic activity by ACE inhibitors is observed after short- and long-term administration. This beneficial effect of reducing sympathetic activity may contribute to the prolongation of life described in the CONSENSUS-Study.

Protective Effect of Stimulated Vasodilating Systems in Heart Failure?

Amelioration of the vicious circle caused by stimulation of vaspressor systems may naturally occur by parallel stimulation of systems with vasodilating activity (Fig. 4) [11]. Among these, the atrial natriuretic peptide (ANP) system has gained the most interest because of its natriuretic and vasodilating properties; however, it remained unclear whether this system would function adequately in heart failure. First results showed markedly elevated levels of this hormone in heart failure. Plasma concentrations of ANP were closely related to atrial pressures and, more precisely, to atrial wall stress [12, 13]. This relationship was observed even in those patients with a long history of heart failure. Hence, heart failure did not prove to be characterized by a lack of a circulating hormone with vasodilating and diuretic properties. Furthermore on a molecular level no resetting phenomenon was observed; close relationships were found between plasma ANP levels and ANP m-RNA in human cardiac atria. Atrial tissue ANP content however was not related either to filling pressures or to plasma levels. The lack of correlation between tissue content and the rate of synthesis indicates a chronic stimulation of atrial ANP production. The activation of synthesis corresponds well with peripheral ANP levels but is not related to intracardiac stores of the hormone. Nonetheless, these results do not imply that this system can cope with additional burdens, for example during physical exercise by patients with heart failure. To further evaluate the capability of this system, two groups of patients were investigated at rest and during exercise: Group 1 consisted of 12 patients with normal values of mean right atrial pressures at rest (i.e. below 5 mm Hg), and group 2 patients had elevated mean right atrial pressures (i.e. above 5 mm Hg) at rest. In this group, mean pulmonary artery pressures and plasma ANP levels were also higher than those of group 1.

During submaximal physical exercise, mean right atrial and mean pulmonary artery pressures rose in parallel in both groups, as did their plasma ANP concentrations. When plasma ANP levels were plotted against mean pulmonary artery pressures, positive linear relationships between both parameters were obtained in

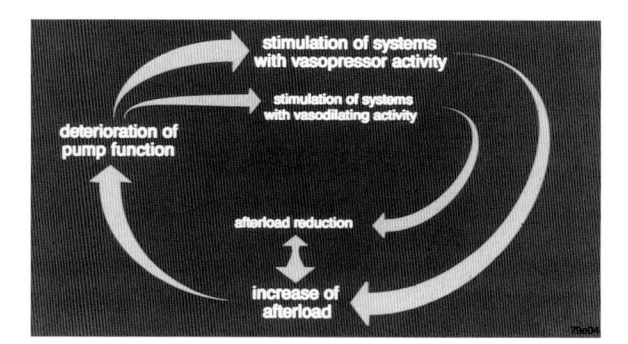

Fig. 4. Amelioration of the vicious circle induced by stimulated vasopressor systems through a parallel stimulation of vasodilator systems. Although inferior in their potency to modulate vasomotor tone in heart failure as compared to the pressor systems, they may exert a small protective effect

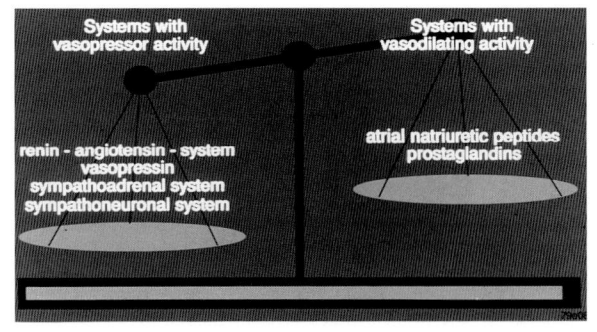

Fig. 5. The number and the strength of systems promoting vasoconstriction in CHF are superior to systems capable of dilating blood vessels. The imbalance between the latter systems is responsible for the elevated afterload in the failing heart syndrome

groups 1 and 2. If anything patients in group 2 appeared to respond a bit more intensively with ANP release to the haemodynamic load than group 1 patients. When the relationships between stimulated ANP release and activation of the sympathetic system were studied, the following observation was made: During physical exercise a stimulated release of both ANP and adrenergic transmitter into the circulation was found in patients with heart failure. The parallel stimulation of the sympathetic and the ANP system in heart failure demonstrates the weakness of the ANP system under these pathophysiological conditions. Although exogenous administration of ANP reduces noradrenaline release, the endogenously stimulated peptide is not effective in suppressing further stimulation of sympathetic activity in heart failure. The imbalance between systems with vasopressor activity and those with vasodilating properties in heart failure contributes to the progression of the disease (Fig. 5); however, the protective effect of endogenous vasodilatory systems – through small – may prevent even more rapid deterioration in the failing heart syndrome.

Malignant Arrhythmias Resulting from Sympathetic Activation, Increased Wall Stress and Electrolyte Imbalance in Heart Failure

The third vicious circle is the activation of sympathetic discharge in combination with an increase in wall stress and electrolyte imbalance (Fig. 6). These represent the trigger mechanisms for aggravating rhythm disturbances [14, 15]. Unfortunately, our therapeutic interventions in the past and the present i.e. administration of digitalis plus diuretics accelerate this vicious circle. The frequent occurrence of tachyarrhythmias further compromises cardiac performance. Antiarrhythmic drugs are not always effective in preventing arrhythmias but they are very often effective in causing further haemodynamic deterioration.

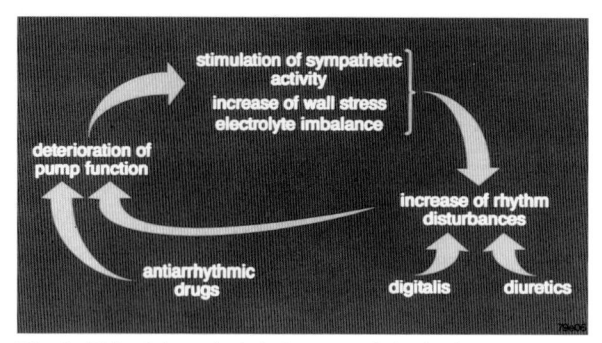

Fig. 6. This vicious circle helps to explain the frequent occurrence of malignant arrhythmias in heart failure. Arrhythmias are facilitated by sympathetic stimulation, increase in wall stress, and electrolyte imbalance. It may be aggravated by common therapy of heart failure, i.e., digitalis and diuretics. Antiarrhythmic drugs very often exhibit proarrhythmic effects in patients with severely impaired pump function and their negative inotropism contributes to a further hemodynamic deterioration

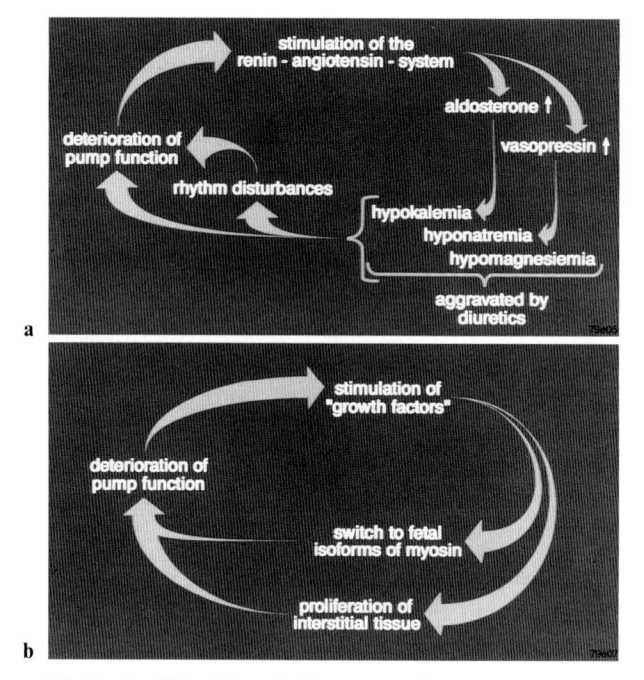

Fig. 7 a, b. This vicious circle represents long-term consequences of the continous stimulation of sympathetic drive and increased activity of the RAS. Both transmitter substances (noradrenaline and angiotensin II) represent growth hormones that act on myocardial tissue composition. Stimulation of α-adrenergic receptors by catecholamines induces a switch to fetal isoforms of myosine in the myocardium. Stimulation of interstitial tissue growth is promoted by angiotensin II and characteristic for dedifferentiation

Stimulation of Growth Factors in Heart Failure: Target for Future Interventions?

All of the vicious circles presented so far have nothing to do with the underlying cause of myocardial failure (Fig. 7). They are only inappropriate responses of the organism to an impaired myocardial pump function. This may be different for the fourth and last vicious circle in heart failure in which the stimulation of the release of several growth factors leads to specific changes in myocardial tissue composition. First there is a switch from adult α myosin heavy chain to the fetal β isoform: β-MHC. Simultaneously, fetal skeletal alpha actin is expressed again. Second, there is stimulated growth of interstitial tissue impeding adequate nutrition and function of cardiac myocytes.

Recent data indicate that catecholamines may act as cardiac growth factors. The α_1 adrenergic receptor is a cardiac growth factor receptor. Its activation by catecholamines induces a switch to synthesis of fetal isoforms of myosin. Stimulation of interstitial tissue growth is promoted by angiotensin II and results in dedifferentation.

Whether re-expression of fetal isogenes represents a beneficial adaptation to haemodynamic overload remains to be elucidated. Progressive interstitial fibrosis, however, is certainly a maladaptation. Future investigations will be directed to identifying the molecular mechanisms of cardiac cell growth in heart failure. This knowledge may provide a basis for manipulating the growth process of myocytes and fibroblasts in the failing human heart.

Conclusion

The severity of heart failure is not precisely described either by the patient's symptoms or by indices of left ventricular pump function. In heart failure, various vicious circles are activated and their activity largely determines the prognosis. An understanding of their mechanism of action will provide the basis for specific therapeutic interventions. Whether these interventions prevent progression of the disease and help to induce regression of maladaptation remains to be determined.

References

1. Applefield MM (1986) Chronic congestive heart failure. Where have we been? Where are we heading? Am J Med 80 (suppl 2B):73–77
2. Dietz R, Waas W, Haass M, Osterziel KJ, Kübler W (1989) Changes in cardiac hormone secretion following acute intravenous administration of enalaprilat in patients with heart failure. 3rd Cardiovascular Pharmacotherapy International Symposium, 15.–19. October, Kyoto, Japan, Abstract Book
3. Halperin JL, Faxon DP, Creager MA, Bass TA, Melidossian CD, Gavras H, Ryan TJ (1982) Coronary hemodynamic effects of angiotensin inhibition by captopril and teprotide in patients with congestive heart failure. Am J Cardiol 50:967–972

4. DeMarco T, Daly PA, Liu M, Kayser S, Parmley W, Chatterjee K (1987) Enalaprilat, a new parenteral angiotensin-converting enzyme inhibitor: rapid changes in systemic and coronary hemodynamics and humoral profile in chronic heart failure. J Am Coll Cardiol 9:1131–1138
5. Magrini F, Shimizu M, Roberts N, Fouad FM, Tarazi RC, Zanchetti A (1987) Converting-enzyme inhibition and coronary blood flow. Circulation 75 (suppl 1):168–174
6. Foult JM, Tavolaro O, Antony I, Nitenberg A (1988) Direct myocardial and coronary effects of enalaprilat in patients with dilated cardiomyopathy: assessment by bilateral intracoronary infusion technique. Circulation 77 (2):337–344
7. Cohn J (1981) Physiological basis of vasodilator therapy for heart failure. Am J Med 71:135–139
8. Osterziel KJ, Dietz R, Kübler W (1989) Bedeutung des sympathischen Nervensystems für die Progression der Herzinsuffizienz. Z Kardiol 78 (suppl 1):100
9. Ludbrook J, Mancia G, Ferrari A, Zanchetti A (1977) The variable-pressure neck-chamber method for studying the carotid baroreflex in man. Clin Sci Mol Med 53:165–171
10. Mancia G, Ferrari A, Gregorini L, Valentini R, Ludbrook J, Zanchetti A (1977) Circulatory reflexes from carotid and extracarotid baroreceptor in man. Circ Res 41:309–315
11. Dietz R, Haass M, Osterziel KJ (1988) Atrial natriuretic factor and arginine vasopressin. In: Cohn J, Mancia G (eds) Failing Heart Syndrome. Series Imperial Chemical Industries PLC, pp 29–44
12. Dietz R, Purgaj J, Lang RE, Schömig A (1986) Pressure dependent release of atrial natriuretic peptide (ANP) in patients with chronic heart disease: does it reset? Klin Wochenschr 64 (suppl VI):42–46
13. Haass M, Dietz R, Fischer Th, Lang RE, Kübler W (1988) Role of right and left atrial dimensions for release of atrial natriuretic peptide in left-sided valvular heart disease and idiopathic dilated cardiomyopathy. Am J Cardiol 62:764–770
14. Bigger JT (1987) Why patients with congestive heart failure die: arrhythmias and sudden cardiac death. Circulation 75 (suppl IV):28–35
15. Francis GS (1986) Development of arrhythmias in the patient with congestive heart failure: pathophysiology, prevalence and prognosis. Am J Cardiol 57:3B–7B

Tissue Renin-Angiotensin Systems in the Pathophysiology of Heart Failure *

A.T. HIRSCH and V.J. DZAU

Circulating Neurohormonal Control Mechanisms in Heart Failure

It is well documented that a reduction in cardiac output elicits compensatory homeostatic responses that are mediated by neurohormonal mechanisms. Activation of the sympathetic nervous system results in systemic vasoconstriction, decreases in renal blood flow and glomerular filtration rate, and an increase in tubular reabsorption of sodium [1]. Activation of the renin-angiotensin system (RAS) contributes further to the increases in vascular tone and sodium avidity. While vasopressin secretion may also be increased during marked reductions in cardiac output, it is unlikely that this hormone contributes significantly to the maintainance of systemic vasoconstriction, as compared to its effects on sodium and water homeostasis [2-4]. The temporal activation of circulating neurohormonal mechanisms are well-illustrated by the study of Watkins et al., in the experimental canine model of cardiac decompensation [5]. In this model, reductions in cardiac output and filling pressure result in the elevations of plasma renin activity and angiotensin II (AII) aldosterone, norepinephrine, and vasopressin levels that are associated with vasoconstriction and sodium retention. However, these circulating neurohormonal mechanisms return toward normal during the compensated stage of heart failure as plasma volume and cardiac stroke volume increase. Thus, in experimental heart failure, circulating neurohormonal mechanisms exhibit a time-dependent response, with acute activation and subsequent normalization during the chronic, compensated phase (Fig. 1). A similar pattern of activation of plasma neurohormones has been observed in patients with heart failure [6]. In patients with mild heart failure or stable disease, plasma renin activity and catecholamine and vasopressin levels are usually normal at rest. Additionally, in animal models of compensated heart failure, such as in rats with coronary ligatures or in dogs during the subacute stage of rapid ventricular pacing, normal or near-normal plasma renin activity and A-II levels have been demonstrated [3, 7, 8]. Nevertheless, chronic angiotensin converting enzyme (ACE) inhibition elicits salutary responses in both patients and animals with stable cardiac dysfunction. The agents inhibiting ACE improve left ventricular

---

* This study was supported by NIH grants HL35610, HL35792, HL35252, HL40210, HL42663, an NIH Specialized Center of Research in Hypertension HL36568, as well as a grant from the Squibb Institute for Medical Research. Dr. A.T. Hirsch is a recipient of an individual NRSA award, F32. HL07702-02.

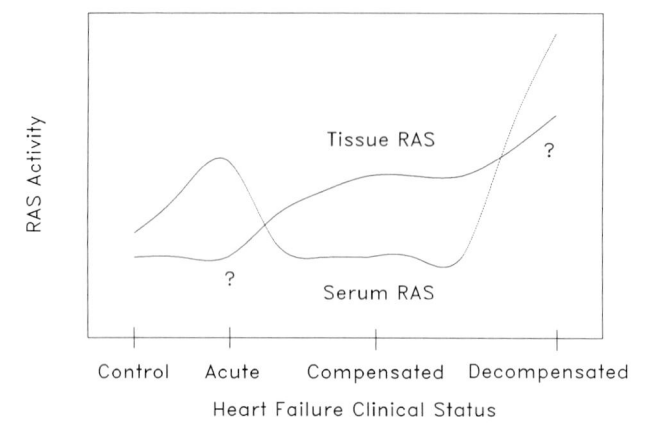

Fig. 1. The relative contributions of the plasma and tissue renin-angiotensin systems (*RAS*) to the natural history of heart failure. Cardiac decompensation likely causes the acute activation of the circulating renin-angiotensin system; the acute response of the tissue RAS is not known (?). During compensated heart failure, local RAS are activated and the circulating RAS activity has been shown to be normal. It is known that the circulating RAS is again activated during decompensated states; further activation of the tissue RAS is presumed (?) is this condition

function, attenuate cardiac remodeling, normalize regional blood flow, and induce renal natriuresis. Overall, morbidity is decreased and survival may be prolonged. We hypothesize that during the compensated phase, the tissue RAS may contribute to the pathophysiology of heart failure. Examination of the role of the tissue RAS in this disease state may also provide insights into the mechanisms mediating the beneficial therapeutic responses to ACE inhibition.

The Tissue RAS in Heart Failure

The circulating peptide hormone, AII, elicits tissue-specific responses at many target organs, including blood vessels, kidney, heart, brain, and adrenal tissues. Recently, an endogenous RAS has been demonstrated in many important tissues. Renin-like enzymic activity, renin substrate, and ACE have been demonstrated at the tissue level using biochemical and immunohistochemical techniques [9–11]. Molecular biological techniques have been used to confirm that both renin and angiotensinogen genes are expressed in many tissues associated with cardiovascular homeostasis, e.g., blood vessels, heart, kidney, brain, and adrenal tissues [12, 13]. In addition, there is evidence for uptake of renin and angiotensinogen by the blood vessel wall [14, 15]. The regulation of the activity of these systems in blood vessels and cardiac and renal tissue has been the focus of our recent investigation. We have proposed that the tissue RAS is activated in pathophysiologic states, such as heart failure, and that local generation of AII contributes to altered tissue function. In this paper, we will review the major tissue RAS that may be involved in the pathophysiology of heart failure.

The Vascular RAS

The existence of renin, angiotensinogen, and AII in blood vessels have been reported by a number of laboratories [16, 17]. The vessel wall distribution of renin has been demonstrated by using anti-renin specific antibody; these studies have demonstrated intense staining throughout the thickness of the aorta, large and smaller arteries, and arterioles, particularly in the endothelial smooth muscle cells [18]. The function of the vascular RAS has been suggested by many studies. Oliver et al. demonstrated that the isolated rat hindlimb artery was capable of generating angiotensin from tetradecapeptide renin-substrate in the absence of exogenous renin [15]. Local angiotensin synthesis is also suggested by the presence of AII in rat plasma 48 h after bilateral nephrectomy, when plasma renin activity is undetectable [19]. Additionally, kinetic analysis of the in vivo arterial-venous angiotensin I (AI) and AII differences in sheep and humans also supports the concept of peripheral arterial AII production [20].

The local synthesis of AII in the blood vessel wall has important physiologic implications. Increased local concentrations of AII may exert a variety of influences on vascular tone (Table 1), and may contribute directly to regional blood flow regulation by activating specific vascular receptors in sensitive regional circulations (e.g., the kidney). Secondly, increased local RAS activity may amplify catecholamine release from noradrenergic nerve endings, thereby increasing local vascular tone in response to sympathetic activation [21–24]. Endothelial prostacyclin synthesis, a third local determinant of vascular tone, may also be influenced by vascular AII formation. The net effect of tissue RAS activity on an individual vascular bed is therefore dependent upon the relative contributions of these tissue, neural, and hormonal mechanisms. In pathophysiologic states in

Table 1. Potential contributions of selected tissue RAS to the pathophysiology of heart failure

Tissue RAS	Potential tissue effect	Pathophysiologic consequences
Cardiac AII	Facilitate adrenergic state	Dysrhythmia induction
	Proto-oncogene expression	Cardiac hypertrophy[a]
	Direct AII cellular effects	Inotropic effect
		Diastolic dysfunction
	Coronary artery vasoconstriction	Subendocardial ischemia
Vascular AII	Decreased conduit vessel compliance and increased arteriolar resistance	Increased afterload[a]
	Venoconstriction	Increased preload[a]
	Renal/Splanchnic vasoconstriction	Regional blood flow redistribution
Renal AII	Proximal tubular Na^+ reabsorption	Increased plasma volume[a]
	Efferent arteriole vasoconstriction	↔, ↑GFR
		↓RBF

[a] These effects would promote myocardial hypertrophy and progressive cardiac dilation.

which the neuroendocrine systems are not activated (e.g., chronic stable heart failure), these local tissue mechanisms may predominate.

Evidence to support the importance of local AII to arteriolar and conduit artery function are derived from experiments involving blockade of renin or angiotensin effects. Longnecker et al. demonstrated that administration of saralasin to spontaneously hypertensive rats resulted in arteriolar vasodilation [25]. The fact that inhibition of the RAS is so efficacious in low-renin hypertensive patients also suggests that a vascular tissue RAS is the locus of angiotensin inhibition. Prolonged infusion of saralasin normalizes blood pressure in the chronic phase of the two-kidney, one-clip model of hypertension [26]. In the chronic phase of hypertension in this model, plasma renin activity is near normal, but vascular renin-angiotensin activity is increased; additionally, increased vascular ACE activity is responsible for the increased vasoconstrictor response to AI infusion [27]. Further evidence to support the contribution of vascular RAS activity to blood pressure control is provided by the data of Unger et al. [28]. In this study, the investigators observed a prolonged hypotensive response after withdrawal of chronically administered ACE inhibitors, despite the immediate return of plasma ACE activity to normal values. These data suggest that inhibition of plasma ACE activity is not essential to elicit a systemic hypotensive response. In fact, sustained inhibition of vascular ACE activity was observed in parallel to the blood pressure response. These data suggest that the inhibition of arteriolar ACE may underlie the antihypertensive effect. In humans, the compliance and diameter of large (brachial and carotid) arteries is increased by ACE inhibition, even at doses that are without a systemic hypotensive response [29, 30]. This latter observation suggests that local vascular RAS activity influences the buffering function of these conduit vessels. This effect of vascular RAS on arterial compliance may result in decreased ventricular afterload when ACE inhibitors are administered in heart failure. Since afterload is an important contributor to ventricular wall stress, the inhibition of vascular ACE may attenuate the progression of cardiac dilatation in heart failure.

The Cardiac RAS

The presence of components of the RAS in the heart have also been demonstrated by enzymatic, biochemical, and molecular biological techniques. Renin enzymic activity has been demonstrated in isolated cardiac myocytes [31]. Cardiac renin mRNA is indistinguishable from renal renin mRNA, and cardiac angiotensinogen mRNA is indistinguishable in sequence from its hepatic counterpart [13, 32, 33]. The presence of ACE in the rat heart has been demonstrated [8, 34, 35]. Recent data suggest that cardiac ACE is located throughout cardiac tissues, but is greatest in the atria, vasculature, conduction system, and cardiac valves (Bruce Jackson, personal communication). The demonstration that conversion of AI to AII by the isolated rat heart provides evidence that this tissue RAS is functionally independent from the circulating RAS [36]. In this ex vivo system, ACE inhibitors prevent angiotensin conversion. Cardiac AII may exert its effects via membrane AII binding sites, whose presence has been confirmed in myocyte cell cultures [37], as well as in human myocardial tissue [38].

The activity of this system can be modulated by various physiologic perturbations. For example, the expressions of both angiotensinogen and renin are increased in the hearts of sodium depleted animals [39]. We have also demonstrated that cardiac and renal renin expressions are selectively increased in response to the infusion of isoproterenol [39]. The dietary sodium restriction, diuretic use, and activated sympathetic nervous system that often accompany clinical heart failure may therefore increase myocardial RAS activity. While increased vascular RAS activity may contribute to the increase in afterload in hypertensive rat models [27, 40], the contribution of cardiac RAS activity in pathophysiologic status has only recently been investigated. We have recently studied cardiac ACE activity in rats with left ventricular hypertrophy induced by aortic banding; in this model, there is a marked rise in cardiac ACE activity and an increase in the cardiac conversion rate of AI to AII [41]. We have also recently demonstrated that cardiac angiotensin-converting enzyme is elevated in the chronic, compensated state of experimental heart failure in the rat [8]. As in stable human disease, plasma renin and serum ACE activities are not elevated during the chronic compensated phase in this animal model. Interestingly, the level of activation of ventricular ACE correlated with the size of myocardial infarction. The increase in right ventricular and interventricular septal ACE activities in rats with experimental heart failure is probably due to the induction of ACE expression with increased local enzyme synthesis; however, the exact stimulus for the induction of cardiac ACE is unclear. In this model of heart failure, Drexler hat also demonstrated induction of the expression of atrial natriuretic factor in the ventricular myocardium in proportion to the extent of myocardial infarction [42]. It is possible that an increase in ventricular dimension and/or wall tension may be a direct stimulus, or that increased myocardial neurosympathetic activity is responsible. It is unlikely that the increased cardiac ACE activity is due to contamination or uptake of serum ACE since cardiac ACE activity (but not serum or other tissue ACE activities) is selectively increased in this rat model.

The increase in cardiac ACE activity in the hypertrophied or failing myocardium may have important pathophysiologic implications. AII may elicit intense coronary artery vasoconstriction; the coronary vasodilatory effect of ACE inhibitors, independent of circulating AII, has been demonstrated in the isolated perfused heart by both Linz and Van Gilst [36, 43]. Locally synthesized cardiac AII may also directly influence cardiac function and metabolism. AII may possess inotropic effects in the failing heart [44–46] or indirectly augment cardiac systolic function via facilitation of norepinephrine release from sympathetic nerve terminals [47, 48]. In the hypertrophied rat myocardium studied as a Langendorf preparation, infusion of AI induces a dose-dependent increase in LV end diastolic pressure; thus, local AII generation may modulate diastolic function in this model. Cardiac angiotensin may also participate in ventricular hypertrophy and remodeling via its growth promoting effects [49]. Indeed, in the hypertrophied isolated heart preparation increased AI to AII conversion was associated with increased expressions of the protooncogenes c-*fos*, c-*myc*, and c-*jun*. These observations may underlie the ability to ACE inhibitors to produce regression of cardiac hypertrophy secondary to chronic hypertension [50]. Thus, the increased cardiac ACE activity and locally synthesized AII may participate in the ventricular remodeling that is ultimately responsible for cardiac dilatation. This enhanced cardiac AII generation may also contribute to the increased ventricular dysrhythmias that are characteristic of advanced cardiac dysfunction.

The Renal RAS in Heart Failure

The presence of a RAS system in the kidney has also been documented by molecular biological, immunocytochemical, and biochemical techniques. Angiotensinogen mRNA in both renal cortex and medulla has been demonstrated [11, 51]. Taugner et al. have demonstrated renin in afferent and efferent arterioles and interlobular arteries by antirenin antiserum staining [52]. Cultured glomerular mesangial cells synthesize renin [53]. In situ hybridization studies have shown that angiotensinogen mRNA is expressed principally in the proximal tubule, while renin mRNA is primarily localized to the juxtaglomerular cells. We have proposed that filtered renin is absorbed into the proximal tubule where it reacts with locally synthesized angiotensinogen to generate AI. The presence of a local renal RAS has important physiologic implications. Proximal tubular ACE converts AI to AII, which may then activate tubular receptors. Cogan et al. showed that AII is a powerful stimulus for sodium reabsorption in the first segment of the proximal tubule [54]. AII also activates Na^+-H^+ exchange and acidifies urine at that site. This intrarenal RAS may also be important in the regulation of sodium homeostasis and glomerular filtration.

As noted above, we have recently observed that experimental heart failure causes renal-specific changes in components of the RAS. In the chronic state after experimental myocardial infarction in the rat, the renal angiotensinogen mRNA level is increased two-fold as compared to sham-operated controls [55]. The magnitude of increase correlated closely with the histopathologic size of the myocardial infarction, implying a relationship with the degree of ventricular dysfunction. This increased renal angiotensinogen expression was tissue specific as extrarenal tissue angiotensinogen mRNA levels were not altered. Similarly, the effect of heart failure on the kidney RAS was selective for this single component of the RAS, as renal renin and ACE activity were unchanged. Interestingly, chronic ACE inhibition with enalapril normalized renal angiotensinogen expression to that of sham-operated control rats, suggesting that angiotensin may have a positive feedback role on angiotensinogen expression in the kidney. Thus, these data may explain why treatment with ACE inhibitors elicits renal vasodilation and natriuresis despite normal activity of the circulatory RAS [56, 57].

Relative Contributions of the Plasma and Tissue RAS

ACE inhibition has been shown to prolong survival in patients with congestive heart failure [58]. Since ACE inhibition has been shown to decrease ventricular volumes in both animal models and humans after myocardial infarction [59–61], it is attractive to presume that these agents will demonstrate sustained efficacy in improving mortality. Thus, the mechanism of action of these pharmacologic agents is important. As reviewed above, data from clinical studies and models of experimental heart failure demonstrate that the plasma RAS is activated in states of acute or decompensated cardiac function. Recently we have demonstrated that cardiac and renal RAS activities are increased in the compensated stage of heart failure at a time when plasma renin angiotensin activity is normal. Therefore, we hypothesize that the plasma RAS serves to maintain circulatory homeostasis during acute and subacute alterations in cardiac output, while changes in tissue RAS contribute to homeostatic responses during chronic sustained impairment of cardiac function (Fig. 1). This concept of a differential contribution of the circulatory and tissue RAS to the pathophysiology of heart failure may have important pharmacologic implications.

Relevance to Pharmacologic Therapy

In as much as local formation of AII in tissues may contribute to abnormalities in vascular, cardiac, and renal function in heart failure, inhibition of these systems is likely to mediate the benefits of pharmacologic therapy in this disease state (Table 1). Thus, in animal models of heart failure and in clinical disease, ACE inhibitors demonstrate efficacy despite normal plasma renin activity. Whereas the acute vasodilatory response to an ACE inhibitor is influenced by the activity of the circulating RAS, the long-term hypotensive response to ACE inhibitors may be more dependent upon inhibition of vascular ACE activity. Vascular ACE inhibition may decrease cardiac preload via venodilation and similarly decrease cardiac afterload via increased conduit artery compliance. The altered regional blood flow in heart failure is also normalized by ACE inhibition. Thus, blockade of AII production by ACE inhibitor also mediates renal vasodilation and elicits natriuresis via ACE blockade at the proximal tubule. The diuretic and natriuretic properties of ACE inhibitors thereby decrease plasma volume and further improve cardiac preload. Inhibition of cardiac angiotensin converting enzyme may improve coronary blood flow, decrease norepinephrine release at cardiac sympathetic nerve terminals, and reduce ventricular dysrhythmias. AII has been demonstrated to promote myocyte growth, and converting-enzyme inhibition has been shown to prevent cardiac hypertrophy and dilatation. Taken together, the inhibition of tissue AII production by chronic ACE inhibition may provide an important mechanism of the beneficial effects of these agents.

Local RAS activity may elicit important end-organ effects; it is attractive to speculate that these systems may explain differential pharmacologic effects of ACE inhibitors. Animal data demonstrate that plasma pharmacokinetics do not predict the tissue half-life of these agents. For example, captopril administration to SHR rats inhibits blood vessel and renal ACE for days longer than its plasma effects [34]. Captopril, fosinopril, and zofenipril produce greater and more prolonged inhibition of SHR rat cardiac ACE after a single oral dose than ramipril and enalapril [62]. Similar disparities in tissue ACE inhibition by various agents have been demonstrated in brain and renal tissue.

Thus, target tissue penetration and/or binding by these agents to converting enzyme may underlie clinically important effects. Neither the pretreatment PRA nor the acute hypotensive response to converting enzyme inhibition predicts long-term efficacy in heart failure patients [63, 64]. It has been suggested that long-acting ACE inhibitors may have greater adverse effects on renal function than short-acting agents [65]. These adverse effects were attributed to more prolonged systemic hypotension than occurred with "shorter-acting" agents. However, equipotent doses may not have been examined. The inability to define tissue-specific ACE inhibition equipotency in clinical trials may also explain, in part, the recent reports of disparate effects of captopril and lisinopril on left ventricular ejection fraction in patients with heart failure [66], or differeing effects of these agents on exercise duration.

In summary, tissue RAS may contribute to the pathophysiology of heart failure via direct myocardial RAS effects, effects on afterload (vascular RAS activity), and effects on preload (vascular and renal tissue RAS activity). ACE inhibition may beneficially improve the prognosis of heart failure via effects on tissue RAS.

References

1. DiBona GF (1977) Neurogenic regulation of renal tubular sodium reabsorption. Am J Physiol 233:173–181
2. Creager MA (1986) The role of vasopressin in congestive heart failure. Heart Failure 2:14–20
3. Hirsch AT, Cant JR, Dzau VJ, Barger AC (1988) Sequential cardiorenal responses to rapid ventricular pacing in the conscious dog. FASEB J 2:A829
4. Paganelli W, Creager MA, Dzau VJ (1986) Cardiac regulation of kidney function. In: Cheung TO (ed) International textbook of cardiology. Gower, London, pp 918–922
5. Watkins IJ, Burton JA, Haber E, Cant JR, Smith FM, Barger AC (1976) The renin-aldosterone system in congestive heart failure in conscious dogs. J Clin Invest 57:1606–1617
6. Dzau VJ, Colucci WS, Hollenberg NK, Williams GH (1981) Relation of the renin-angiotensin-aldosterone system to clinical state in congestive heart failure. Circulation 63:645–651
7. Hodsman GP, Kohzuki M, Howes LG, Sumithran E, Tsunoda K, Johnston CI (1988) Neurohormonal responses to chronic myocardial infarction in rats. Circulation 78:376–381
8. Hirsch AT, Talsness C, Lage A, Dzau VJ (1989) The effect of experimental myocardial infarction and chronic captopril treatment on plasma and tissue angiotensin converting-enzyme activity. Clin Res 37:266A (abstract)
9. Deboben A, Inagami T, Ganten G (1983) Tissue renin. In: Genest J, Kuchel O, Hamet P (eds) Hypertension, 2nd edn. McGraw-Hill, New York, pp 194–209
10. Philips MI, Stenstrom B (1985) Angiotensin II in rat brain comigrates with authentic angiotensin II in high pressure liquid chromatography. Circ Res 56:212–219
11. Dzau VJ, Ellison KE, Brody T, Ingelfinger J, Pratt RE (1987) A comparative study of the distributions of renin and angiotensinogen messenger ribonucleic acids in rat and mouse tissues. Endocrinology 120:2334–2338
12. Field LS, McGowen RA, Dickenson DP, Gross KW (1984) Tissue and gene specificity of mouse renin expression. Hypertension 6:597–603
13. Lynch KR, Simnad VT, Ben-Ari ET, Maniatis R, Zinn K, Garrison JC (1986) Localization of preangiotensinogen messenger RNA sequences in the rat brain. Hypertension 8:540–543
14. Loudon M, Bing RF, Thurston H, Swales JD (1983) Arterial wall uptake of renal renin and blood pressure control. Hypertension 5:629–634
15. Oliver JA, Sciacca RR (1984) Local generation of angiotensin II as a mechanism of regulation of peripheral vascular tone in the rat. J Clin Invest 74:1247–1251
16. Dzau VJ, Gibbons GH (1987) Autocrine-paracrine mechanisms of vascular myocytes in hypertension. Am J Cardiol 60:991–1031

17. Rosenthal JH, Pfeiffer B, Mecheilor ML, Pschorr J, Jacob ICM, Dahlheim H (1984) Investigations of components of the renin-angiotensin system in rat vascular tissue. Hypertension 6:383–390
18. Molteni A, Dzau VJ, Fallon JT, Haber E (1984) Monoclonal antibodies as probes of renin gene expression. Circulation 70 [Suppl II]:II-196
19. Aguirela G, Schirer A, Baukai A, Gatt KJ (1981) Circulating angiotensin II and adrenal receptors after nephrectomy. Nature 289:507–509
20. Campbell DJ (1985) The site of angiotensin production. J Hypertens 3:730–737
21. Malik KU, Masjletti A (1976) Facilitation of adrenergic transmission by locally generated angiotensin II in rat mesenteric arteries. Circ Res 60(3):422–428
22. Zimmerman BG (1981) Adrenergic facilitation by angiotensin. Does it serve a physiological function? Clin Sci 60:343–348
23. Kawasaki H, Cline WH Jr, Su C (1984) Involvement of the vascular renin-angiotensin system in beta adrenergic receptor-mediated facilitation of vascular neurotransmission in spontaneously hypertensive rats. J Pharmacol Exp Ther 231:23–32
24. Nakamura M, Jackson EK, Inagami T (1986) Beta adrenoreceptor mediated release of angiotensin II from mesenteric arteries. Am J Physiol 250:H144–H148
25. Longnecker DI, Durcus MI, Donovan KR, Miller ED, Peach MJ (1984) Saralasin dilates arterioles in SHR but not WKY rats. Hypertension I [Suppl 1]:106–110
26. Riegger AJG, Lever AF, Miller JA, Morton JJ, Slack B (1977) Correction of renal hypertension in the rat by prolonged infusion of saralasin. Lancet 2:1317–1319
27. Okamura T, Miyazcki M, Inagemi T, Toda N (1986) Vascular renin-angiotensin system in two-kidney, one clip hypertensive rates. Hypertension 8:560–565
28. Unger T, Ganten D, Lang RE, Scholkens VA (1985) Is tissue converting inhibition a determinant of the antihypertensive efficacy of converting enzyme inhibitors? Studies with two different compounds. Hoe 398 and MD 421 in spontaneously hypertensive rats. J Cardiovasc Pharmacol 7:36–41
29. Simon ACH, Levenson JA, Bouther JI, Safar ME (1984) Comparison of oral MK 421 and propranolol in mild to moderate hypertension and their effects on arterial and venous vessels of the forearm. Am J Cardiol 53:781–783
30. Dzau VJ, Safar MI (1988) Large conduit arteries in hypertension; role of the vascular renin angiotensin system. Circulation 77:947–954
31. Dzau VJ, Re RN (1987) Evidence for the existence of renin in the heart. Circulation 73 [Suppl I]:134–136
32. Piccini N, Knopf JL, Gross KW (1982) A DNA polmorphism, consistent with gene duplications, correlates with renin levels in the mouse submaxillary gland. Cell 30:205
33. Ohkubo H, Nakayama K, Tanaka T, Nakanishi S (1986) Tissue distribution of rat angiotensinogen mRNA and structural analysis of its heterogeneity. J Biol Chem 261:319–323
34. Cohen L, Kurz KD (1982) Angiotensin converting enzyme inhibition in tissues from spontaneously hypertensive rats after treatment with captopril or MK-421. J Pharmacol Exp Ther 220:63–69
35. Unger T, Demmert G, Flect T (1984) Role of tissue converting enzyme inhibition for the antihypertensive action of Hoe 498 and MK 421 in spontaneously hypertensive rats. Naunyn Schmiedebergs Arch Pharmacol 325 [Suppl]:216
36. Linz W, Scholkens BA, Han YI (1986) Beneficial effects of the converting enzyme inhibition, ramipril in ischemic rat hearts. J Cardiovasc Pharmacol 8 [Suppl 10]:591–599
37. Rogers TB, Gaa S, Allen IS (1986) Identification and characterization of functional angiotensin II receptors on cultured heart myocytes. J Pharmacol Exp Ther 236:438–444
38. Urata H, Healy B, Stewart RW, Bumpus FM, Husain A (1989) Angiotensin II receptors in normal and failing human hearts. J Clin Endocrinol Metab 69:54–66
39. Dzau VJ, Ellison KE, Ouellette AJ (1985) Expression and regulation of renin in the mouse heart. Clin Res 33:181A (abstract)
40. Assad MM, Antonaccio MJ (1982) Vascular wall renin in spontaneously hypertensive rats: potential relevance to hypertension maintenance and antihypertensive effect of captopril. Hypertension 4:487–493
41. Lorell BH, Schunkert H, Grice WN, Tang SS, Abstein CS, Dzau VJ (1989) Alteration in cardiac angiotensin converting enzyme activity in pressure overload hypertrophy. Circulation 80 [Suppl II]:II-297 (abstract)

42. Drexler H, Hanze J, Finch M, Lu W, Just H, Lang RE (1989) Atrial natriuretic peptide in a rat model of cardiac failure. Circulation 79:620–633
43. Van Gilst WH, deGraeff PA, Wessling H, deLangen CDJ (1987) Reduction of reperfusion arrhythmias in the ischemic isolated rat heart by angiotensin converting enzyme inhibitors: a comparison of captopril, enalapril and HOE 498. J Cardiovasc Pharmacol 9:254–255
44. Baker KM, Khosla MC (1986) Cardiac and vascular actions of decapeptide angiotensin analogs. J Pharmacol Exp Ther 239:790–796
45. Koch-Weser J (1965) Nature of the inotropic action of angiotensin on ventricular myocardium. Circ Res 16:230–237
46. Koch-Weser J (1964) Myocardial actions of angiotensin II. Circ Res 14:337–344
47. Ziogas J, Story DF, Rand MJ (1985) Effects of locally generated AII on noradrenergic transmission in guinea pig isolated atria. Eur J Pharmacol 106:11–18
48. Ziang J, Linz W, Becker H, Ganten D, Lang RE, Schoelkens B, Unger T (1984) Effects of converting enzyme inhibitors: ramipril and enalapril on peptide action and sympathetic neurotransmission in the isolated rat heart. Eur J Pharmacol 113:215–223
49. Naftilan AJ, Pratt RJ, Eldridge CS, Lin HL, Dzau VJ (1989) Angiotensin II induces c-*fos* expression in smooth muscle via transcriptional control. Hypertension 13:706–711
50. Tarazi RC, Fouad FM (1984) Reversal of cardiac hypertrophy. Hypertension 6 [Suppl III]: III-140–III-145
51. Ingelfinger JR, Pratt RE, Ellison K, Dzau VJ (1986) Sodium regulation of angiotensinogen mRNA expression in rat kidney cortex and medulla. J Clin Invest 78:1311–1315
52. Taugner R, Hackenthal E, Helmchen U, Ganten D, Kugler P, Marin-Grez M, Nobiling R, Unger T, Lockwald I, Keilbach R (1982) The intrarenal renin-angiotensin system. An immunocytochemical study on the localization of renin, angiotensinogen, converting enzyme, and the angiotensins in the kidney of mouse and rat. Klin Wochenschr 60:1218–1222
53. Dzau VJ, Kreisberg JI (1986) Cultured glomerular mesangial cells contain renin: influence of calcium and isoproterenol. J Cardiovasc Pharmacol 8 [Suppl 10]:S6–S10
54. Liu FY, Cogan MG (1987) Angiotensin II: a potent regulator of acidification in the rat early proximal convoluted tubule. J Clin Invest 80:273–275
55. Schunkert H, Hirsch AT, Mankadi S, Talsness C, Dzau VJ (1989) Renal angiotensinogen gene expression in experimental heart failure: effect of angiotensin converting-enzyme inhibition. Clin Res 37:584A
56. Hostetter TH, Pfeffer JM, Pfeffer MA, Dworkin LD, Braunwald E, Brenner BM (1983) Cardiorenal hemodynamics and sodium excretion in rats with myocardial infarction. Am J Physiol 245:H98–H103
57. Ichikawa I, Pfeffer JM, Pfeffer MA, Hostetter TH, Brenner BM (1984) Role of angiotensin II in the altered renal function of congestive heart failure. Circ Res 55:669–675
58. The CONSENSUS Trial Study Group (1987) Effects of enalapril on mortality in severe heart failure. N Engl J Med 316:1429–1431
59. Pfeffer JM, Pfeffer MA, Braunwald E (1985) Influence of chronic captopril therapy on the infarcted left ventricle of the rat. Circ Res 57:84–95
60. Pfeffer MA, Lamas GA, Vaughn DE, Parisi AF, Braunwald E (1988) Effect of captopril on progressive ventricular dilatation after anterior myocardial infarction. N Engl J Med 319:80–86
61. Sharpe N, Murphy J, Smith H, Hannan S (1988) Treatment of patients with symptomless left ventricular dysfunction after myocardial infarction. Lancet 1(8580):255–259
62. Cushman DW, Wang FL, Fung WC, Harvey CM, DeForrest JM (1989) Differentiation of angiotensin-converting enzyme (ACE) inhibitors by their selective inhibition of ACE in physiologically important target organs. Am J Hypertens 2:294–306
63. Massie BM, Kramer BL, Topic N (1984) Lack of relationship between the short-term hemodynamic effects of captopril and subsequent clinical responses. Circulation 69:1135–1141
64. Creager MA, Faxon DP, Halperin SL et al. (1982) Determinants of clinical response and survival in patients with congestive heart failure treated with captopril. Am Heart J 104:1147–1153
65. Packer M, Lee WH, Yushak M, Medina N (1981) Comparison of captopril and enalapril in patients with severe chronic heart failure. N Engl J Med 315:847–853
66. Giles TG, Katz R, Sullivan JM, Wolfson P et al. (1989) Short- and long-acting angiotensin converting enzyme inhibitors: a randomized trial of lisinopril versus captopril in the treatment of congestive heart failure. J Am Coll Cardiol 13:1240–1247

Evaluation of the Severity of Ventricular Rhythm Disturbances: Value of Electrophysiological Testing and Recording of Late Potentials

L. SEIPEL, G. BREITHARDT, and M. BORGGREFE

Introduction

Sudden death is one of the major risks in patients suffering from coronary heart disease especially after myocardial infarction. In most instances this final event is caused by ventricular tachyarrhythmias. Many studies have shown that ventricular premature beats are the harbingers of sudden death in these patients [1]. The prerequisite for the induction of ventricular tachyarrhythmias is the arrhythmogenic electrophysiological substrate. The presence of an arrhythmogenic substrate is, however, not sufficient to develop ventricular tachycardia. Instead, some additional factors (such as ventricular premature beats) are necessary to initiate a reentrant tachycardia. Ventricular premature beats can be recorded by Holter monitoring and exercise tests. However, they have been shown to have a low predictive value for sudden death [2, 3]. The presence or absence of an arrhythmogenic substrate can be assessed by means of programmed stimulation (ventricular "vulnerability"). Of course, the fibrillation threshold cannot be measured in man. However, in experimental studies a good correlation between the fibrillation threshold and repetitive ventricular responses was found [4].

Recently, noninvasive recording of ventricular late potentials became possible. Late potentials originate from areas of previous myocardial infarction that may leave a zone of abnormal ventricular myocardium as a potential site of origin of ventricular tachycardia. Thus, this new technique may provide additional information on the presence of an arrhythmogenic substrate.

Patients and Methods

In a prospective study, programmed ventricular stimulation and non-invasive recording of late potentials were performed in two different groups of patients. Group 1 consisted of patients who were referred to coronary angiography; patients in group 2 were drawn from survivors of acute myocardial infarction (Table 1). None of these patients had experienced ventricular tachycardia, fibrillation, or syncope spontaneously before.

The stimulation protocol included the introduction of single and double ventricular extrastimuli during sinus rhythm and paced ventricular rhythm at rates of 120–180 beats per minute [5]. The arbitrary endpoint of the stimulation proto-

Table 1. Patients with coronary artery disease examined by signal averaging and by programmed ventricular stimulation. (From [8])

	Signal averaging	Ventricular stimulation	Both
Total number of patients	665	428	379
Number of patients ≤months after myocardial infarction	314	154	132

col was the induction of a nonsustained ventricular tachycardia defined as four or more consecutive ventricular echo beats. In a previous retrospective analysis, we were able to show that four echo beats was a good discriminating point [6]. In addition, four or more consecutive beats are very unlikely to be due to an bundle branch reentry, which is considered as a physiological phenomenon.

Late potentials were detected by the signal averaging technique from the surface ECG using bipolar leads. The signal was preamplified, bandpass filtered (100–300 Hz, 6 db/octave) and digitally averaged (Princeton Applied Research, Signal Averager Model 4202) [7]. In addition, 24-h Holter monitoring recording, echocardiography, and in most instances (404 of 665 patients) angiocardiography were performed.

Results

In 188 patients (43.9%) the stimulation protocol was terminated because of the induction of nonsustained ventricular tachycardias of four or more ventricular beats. In 45 patients (10.5%) either sustained ventricular tachycardia or ventricular fibrillation was induced. Patients with a history of a myocardial infarction showed an abnormal response in 147 of 279 cases (52.9%). In patients studied 6 weeks after acute myocardial infarction ventricular tachycardia was induced in 31 of 154 cases (20.1%) [8].

The relationship between the results of programmed ventricular stimulation and left ventricular function is shown in Fig. 1. The prevalence of abnormal responses was significantly higher in patients with left ventricular contraction abnormalities (50.8%) as compared to patients with normal left ventricular function (19.2%). An abnormal response was more often observed in patients with anterior than with inferior infarction. In addition, sustained ventricular tachycardia was induced mostly in patients with hypokinesia or dyskinesia of the left ventricle [8].

Late potentials were found in 39.1% (260/665) of the total group of patients. In patients studied within 6 months after myocardial infarction, the prevalence of late potentials was higher (46%) than in those without a history of myocardial infarction (25%). Especially the occurrence of late potentials of long duration (≥ 40 ms) was more frequent in the former group (13.7%) than in the latter (3.4%). Figure 2 shows the correlation of late potentials to left ventricular con-

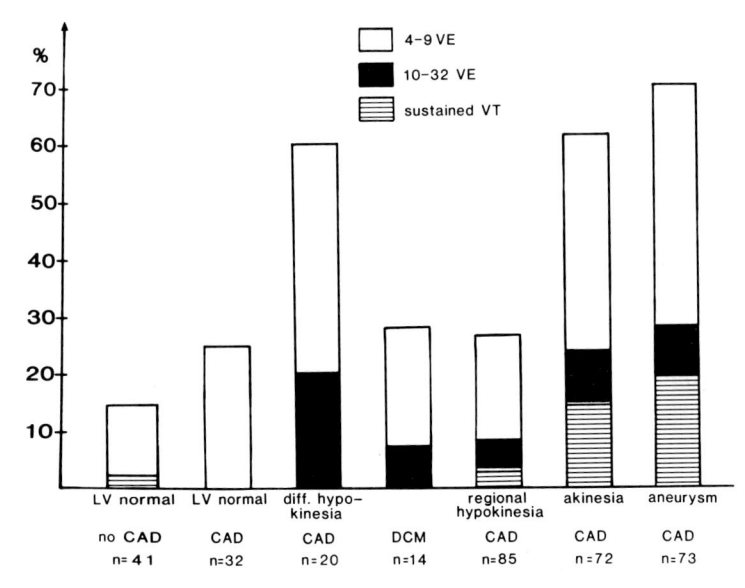

Evaluation of the Severity of Ventricular Rhythm Disturbances

Fig. 1. Correlation between the results of programmed ventricular stimulation and left ventricular function in 337 patients without spontaneous ventricular tachycardia (*VT*) or fibrillation. *VE* = Ventricular echo beats induced by programmed pacing; *CAD* = coronary artery disease; *DCM* = dilated cardiomyopathy

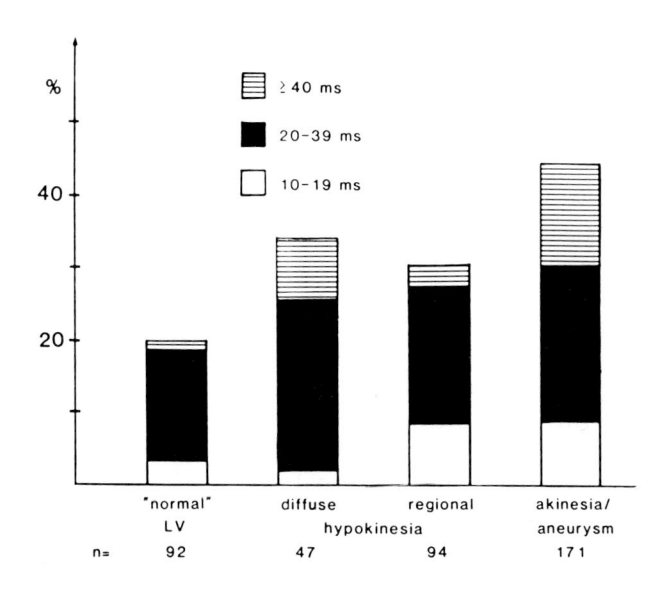

Fig. 2. Correlation between the presence and duration of late potentials and left ventricular function. Although late potentials of a duration between 20 and 39 ms were present in all four groups, those of 40 ms or more were significantly more frequent in patients with diffuse left ventricular hypokinesia, akinesia, or aneurysm

traction abnormalities. They were significantly more frequent in subjects with hypokinesia or aneurysm. This holds true especially for late potentials of long duration (≥ 40 ms) [9].

As shown above, there was a significant correlation between left ventricular function, on the one hand, and the presence of late potentials and abnormal repetitive responses, on the other. In contrast, late potentials and the results of programmed ventricular stimulation were less closely associated [10].

In contrast, the findings of the 24-h monitoring showed no close correlation neither to ventricular vulnerability nor to the prevalence of late potentials. In many patients there was a marked discrepancy between the inducibility of even sustained ventricular tachycardia and the presence of ventricular arrhythmias during Holter monitoring. Although the prevalence of late potentials significantly increased with increasing number of spontaneous premature beats, late potentials of long duration (≥ 40 ms) were not significantly correlated with spontaneous ventricular arrhythmias [8].

Prognostic Significance

In patients with late potentials, sudden death was about three times more frequent than in those without (3.1% versus 0.95%). In the overall group, the predictive value of late potentials was 5.7%, whereas it was 9.2% in patients studied within 6 weeks after myocardial infarction. The predictive value was markedly higher (15.4%) in patients with late potentials of long duration (≥ 40 ms) [11].

There was no correlation between the occurrence of sudden death during follow-up and the results of programmed ventricular stimulation. However, all patients who subsequently developed sustained ventricular tachycardia had an abnormal response, whereas no patients with normal responses during pacing developed a sustained ventricular tachyarrhythmia [8]. This means there was a high number of false-positive results but no false-negative finding. Figure 3 shows the latest results of the follow up of the patients investigated within 6 weeks after acute myocardial infarction. Those with normal repetitive response to programmed ventricular stimulation and no late potentials were nearly eventfree. Patients with only an abnormal response to programmed stimulation and no late potentials or vice verse had about the same good prognosis as far as sudden death or arrhythmic events were concerned. In contrast, patients with an abnormal ventricular "vulnerability" and late potentials had a much higher incidence of these events during follow-up. In patients investigated shortly after acute myocardial infarction, the results of stimulation and averaging had a highly predictive value as far as the spontaneous occurrence of ventricular tachycardia was concerned. Patients with late potentials of long duration (≥ 40 ms) in whom a ventricular tachycardia of relatively slow rate (<270 bpm) could be induced, had a 50% probability to experience spontaneous ventricular tachycardia VT during follow-up [12].

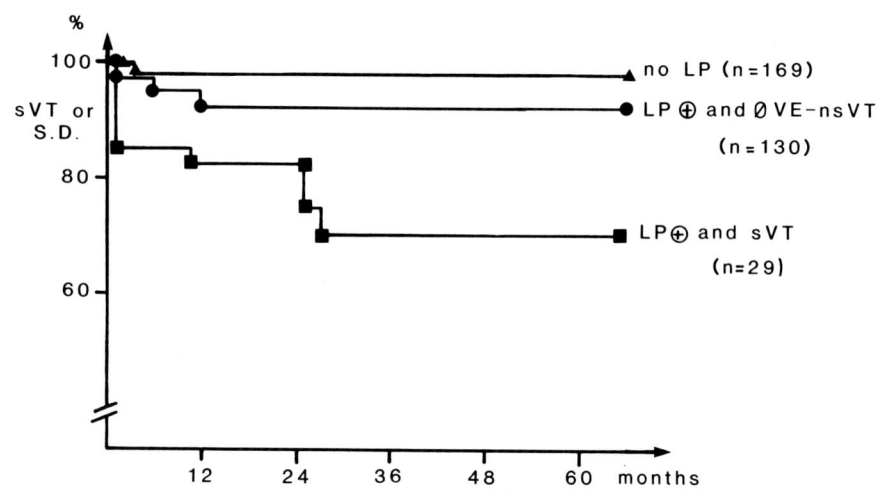

Fig. 3. Prognostic significance of ventricular late potentials (*LP*) and the results of programmed ventricular stimulation after acute myocardial infarction (*MI*). LP⊕ = LP present; ∅VE−ns VT = absence of inducible ventricular echo beats or nonsustained ventricular tachycardia. Patients with LP and inducible sustained VT had a significantly higher incidence of spontaneous VT (*sVT*) or sudden death (*SD*) during follow-up

Discussion

Noninvasive recording of late potentials and ventricular "vulnerability" as assessed by programmed ventricular stimulation have a poor predictive value as far as sudden death during follow-up is concerned. However, in the present study there was a much better correlation between the presence or absence of ventricular late potentials and the results of programmed stimulation to the spontaneous occurrence of ventricular tachycardia. In patients investigated early after acute myocardial infarction, these methods enabled us to characterize a highly endangered subgroup in whom preventive therapy may be justified.

The results of other investigations on the prognostic significance of late potentials are difficult to compare because of different recording techniques, different endpoints, and different patient populations. However, the available data suggest a potential predictive value of late potentials in assessing prognosis after myocardial infarction [13–15]. Late potentials are an important prognostic parameter in the combination with other predictive methods such as Holter monitoring, exercise test, and analysis of left ventricular function [16–19]. In addition, noninvasive recording of late potentials can identify (together with other parameters) a propensity to the induction of monomorphic ventricular tachycardia by programmed pacing in patients after myocardial infarction [20–25]. Therefore, signal averaging respresents a noninvasive technique which might be useful as a screening method for selection of patients for programmed ventricular stimulation.

The results of programmed ventricular stimulation of different groups are difficult to compare because of different stimulation protocols, different endpoints of stimulation, and different endpoints during follow-up. In our study and in studies by several other authors [26-28] the occurrence of sudden death could not be predicted on the basis of programmed stimulation. In contrast, other investigators observed sudden death in a high percentage of patients with abnormal response to programmed stimulation [29, 30]. In our study and in that of Richards et al. [30] and that of Bhandari et al. [26] the inducibility of sustained ventricular tachycardia (but not ventricular fibrillation) identified a group with an arrhythmic event rate between 10% and 20%. Other studies did not report any episode of sustained ventricular tachycardia during follow-up [27-29].

Denniss et al. [31] compared the results of programmed stimulation and signal averaging in a group of patients after myocardial infarction in a prospective fashion. They found a significant correlation between the presence of delayed potentials and the ability to induce ventricular tachycardia. Both parameters were found to predict a significant risk of sudden death or sustained ventricular tachycardia during follow-up with a high sensitivity but low specifity. When both delayed potentials and inducible ventricular tachycardias were present, the predictive value was 33%, that of the negative tests 93%.

Conclusion

Signal averaging and programmed ventricular stimulation appear to be new promising techniques for the identification of patients at risk of ventricular tachyarrhythmias. Which method is most appropriate for risk stratification after myocardial infarction remains to be established. Due to a large proportion of false-positive results obtained with each method, it seems unlikely that either of them will be sufficient to assess the risk of the individual patients. However, a negative test result may identify patients at low risk. A multivariant statistical approach taking into account the results of all presently available noninvasive techniques may be helpful to characterize a subset of highly endangered patients in whom invasive stimulation may be indicated. This stepwise approach may be helpful in the future to predict the risk of the individual patients. This risk stratification may form a basis for medical or nonmedical antiarrhythmic prophylactic interventions in asymptomatic patients after myocardial infarction to prevent arrhythmogenic complications.

References

1. Moss AJ (1980) Clinical significance of ventricular arrhythmias in patients with and without coronary artery disease. Prog Cardiovasc Dis 23:33-52
2. Armstrong WF, McHenry PL (1985) Ambulatory electrocardiographic monitoring: can we predict sudden death? J Am Coll Cardiol 5:13B-16B

3. Kostis JB, Byington R, Friedman LM, Goldstein S, Furberg C (1987) Prognostic significance of ventricular ectopic activity in survivors of acute myocardial infarction. J Am Coll Cardiol 10:237–242
4. Matta RJ, Verrier R, Lown B (1976) The repetitive extrasystole as an index of vulnerability to ventricular fibrillation. Am J Physiol 230:1461
5. Abendroth RR, Breithardt G, Blese HP, Yeh HL, Seipel L (1981) Häufigkeit, Reproduzierbarkeit und prognostische Bedeutung ventrikulärer Echoschläge bei Patienten mit und ohne koronare Herzkrankheit. Z Kardiol 70:889–894
6. Breithardt G, Seipel L, Meyer T, Abendroth RR (1982) Prognostic significance of repetitive ventricular response during programmed ventricular stimulation. Am J Cardiol 49:693–698
7. Breithardt G, Becker R, Seipel L, Abendroth RR, Ostermeyer J (1981) Non-invasive detection of late potentials in man – a new marker for ventricular tachycardia. Eur Heart J 2:1–11
8. Breithardt G, Borggrefe M, Haerten K, Seipel L (1986) Value of electrophysiologic testing, recording of late potentials by averaging techniques and Holter monitoring for the identification of high risk patients after acute myocardial infarction. In: Kulbertus HE (ed) Medical management of cardiac arrhythmias. Churchill Livingstone, Edinburgh, p 228–245
9. Breithardt G, Borggrefe M, Karbenn U, Abendroth RR, Yeh HL, Seipel L (1982) Prevalence of late potentials in patients with and without ventricular tachycardia: correlation with angiographic findings. Am J Cardiol 49:1932–1937
10. Breithardt G, Borggrefe M, Quantius B, Karbenn U, Seipel L (1983) Ventricular vulnerability assessed by programmed ventricular stimulation in patients with and without late potentials. Circulation 68:275–281
11. Breithardt G, Schwarzmaier J, Borggrefe M, Haerten K, Seipel L (1983) Prognostic significance of late ventricular potentials after acute myocardial infarction. Eur Heart J 4:487–495
12. Breithardt G, Broggrefe M (1986) Pathophysiological mechanisms and clinical significance of ventricular late potentials. Eur Heart J 7:364–385
13. Denniss AR, Richards DA, Cody DV, Russell PA, Young AA, Ross DL, Uther JB (1987) Correlation between signal-averaged electrocardiogram and programmed stimulation in patients with and without spontaneous ventricular tachyarrhythmias. Am J Cardiol 59:586–590
14. von Leiter ER, Oeff M, Loock D, Jahns B, Schröder R (1983) Value of non-invasively detected delayed ventricular depolarization to predict prognosis in post myocardial infarction patients (abstr). Circulation 68 [Suppl III]:831
15. Zimmermann M, Adamec R, Simonin P, Richez J (1985) Prognostic significance of ventricular late potentials in coronary artery disease. Am Heart J 109:725–732
16. Cripps T, Bennet D, Camm J, Ward D (1988) Prospective evaluation of clinical assessment, exercise testing and signal-averaged electrocardiogram in predicting outcome after acute myocardial infarction. Am J Cardiol 62:995–999
17. Cripps T, Bennet ED, Camm AJ, Ward DE (1988) High gain signal averaged electrocardiogram combined with 24 hour monitoring in patients early after myocardial infarction for bedside prediction of arrhythmic events. Br Heart J 60:181–187
18. Gomes JA, Winters SL, Stewart D, Horowitz S, Milner M, Barreca P (1987) A new non-invasive index to predict sustained ventricular tachycardia and sudden death in the first year after myocardial infarction: based on signal-averaged electrocardiogram, radionuclide ejection fraction and Holter monitoring. J Am Coll Cardiol 10:349–357
19. Kuchar DL, Thorburn CW, Sammel NL (1987) Prediction of serious arrhythmic events after myocardial infarction: signal-averaged electrocardiogram, Holter monitoring and radionuclide ventriculography. J Am Coll Cardiol 9:531–538
20. Borbola J, Ezri MD, Denes P (1988) Correlation between the signal-averaged electrocardiogram and electrophysiologic study findings in patients with coronary artery disease and sustained ventricular tachycardia. Am Heart J 115:816–824
21. Buxton AE, Simson MB, Falcone RA, Marchlinski FE, Doherty JU, Josephson ME (1987) Results of signal-averaged electrocardiography and electrophysiologic study in patients with non-sustained ventricular tachycardia after healing of acute myocardial infarction. Am J Cardiol 60:80–85

22. Lindsay BD, Ambos HD, Schechtman KB, Cain ME (1986) Improved selection of patients for programmed ventricular stimulation by frequency analysis of signal-averaged electrocardiograms. Circulation 73:675–683
23. Nalos PC, Gang ES, Mandel WJ, Ladenheim ML, Lass Y, Peter T (1987) The signal-averaged electrocardiogram as a screening test for inducibility of sustained ventricular tachycardia in high risk patients: a prospective study. J Am Coll Cardiol 9:539–548
24. Turitto G, Fontaine JM, Ursell SN, Cares EB, Henkin R, El-Sherif N (1988) Value of the signal-averaged electrocardiogram as a predictor of the results of programmed stimulation in nonsustained ventricular tachycardia. Am J Cardiol 61:1272–1278
25. Winters SL, Stewart D, Gomes JA (1987) Signal averaging of the surface QRS complex predicts inducibility of ventricular tachycardia in patients with syncope of unknown origin: a prospective study. J Am Coll Cardiol 10:775–781
26. Bhandari AK, Hong R, Kotlweski A, McIntosh N, Au P, Sankooriskal A, Rhaimtoola S (1989) Prognostic significance of programmed ventricular stimulation in survivors of acute myocardial infarction. Br Heart J 61:410–416
27. Marchlinski FE, Buxton AE, Waxman HL, Josephson ME (1983) Identifying patients at risk of sudden death after myocardial infarction. Value of the response to programmed stimulation, degree of ventricular ectopic activity and severity of left ventricular dysfunction. Am J Cardiol 52:1190–1196
28. Santarelli P, Bellocci F, Lperfido F, Mazzari M, Mongiardo R, Montenero AS, Manzoli U, Denes P (1985) Ventricular arrhythmias induced by programmed ventricular stimulation after myocardial infarction. Am J Cardiol 55:391–394
29. Hamer A, Vohra J, Hunt D, Sloman G (1982) Prediction of sudden death by electrophysiologic studies in high risk patients surviving acute myocardial infarction. Am J Cardiol 50:223–229
30. Richards DA, Cody DV, Dennis AR, Russel PA, Young AA, Uther JB (1983) Ventricular electrical instability: a predictor of death after myocardial infarction. Am J Cardiol 51 (1983) 75–80
31. Denniss RA, Richards DA, Cody DV, Russel PA, Young AA, Cooper MJ, Ross DL, Uther JB (1986) Prognostic significance of ventricular tachycardia and fibrillation induced at programmed stimulation and delayed potentials detected on the signal-averaged electrocardiograms of survivors of acute myocardial infarction. Circulation 74:731–745

II Approaches to Treatment

Hemodynamic Approach

Editorial:
How to Treat – The Hemodynamic Approach

K. Kochsiek

The prognosis of patients with congestive heart failure can be estimated by clinical symptomatology, left ventricular volume and ejection fraction, complex ventricular arrhythmias, and neuroendocrine activation. The cause of heart failure may be biochemical abnormalities of the myocytes responsible for the depressed contractility, which may involve alterations in the receptor population and regulatory proteins, changes in the properties of the sarcolemma and sarcoplasmatic reticulum, and unfavourable alterations of mitochondrial function. The structural basis of the ventricle is also influenced by changes in the non-myocyte compartment, the interstitium and intramural coronary vasculature. Remodeling of the existing fibrillar collagen network and disproportionate accumulation of collagen in the interstitium and around intramyocardial coronary arteries may have important implications for ventricular function, influencing the geometry of the ventricle and diastolic and systolic myocardial stiffness. A third important factor in heart failure, especially with regard to exercise capacity, is blood flow to the vasculature of exercising skeletal muscle, which is reduced by several factors the nature of which is not precisely defined. The most promising therapeutic approach to congestive heart failure is use of angiotensin converting enzyme inhibitors, which due to their multiple sites of action interfere with some of the above-mentioned mechanisms, thereby significantly improving exercise capacity, well-being, and prognosis of patients with heart failure. Until now, there have been no favourable therapeutic modalities for correcting contractility abnormalities of the myocardium and increasing the exercise capacity and prognosis, except for digitalis.

Structural Basis of Left Ventricular Dysfunction: Role of Collagen Network Remodeling and Potential Therapeutic Interventions*

M. A. Silver and K. T. Weber

Introduction

Left ventricular hypertrophy is the primary risk factor associated with the appearance of symptomatic heart failure [1]. Why hypertrophic growth of the myocardium would be adaptive in a weight lifter, fostering enhanced cardiac performance during elevations in arterial pressure associated with isometric exercise, and pathologic in the patient with hypertension, is unclear. In seeking to identify the pathogenetic mechanisms responsible for pathologic hypertrophy, basic and applied scientists have hoped to unravel this puzzle. As an outgrowth of this investigation, important insights into the contractile process of cardiac muscle have emerged while potential biochemical abnormalities that would account for impaired ventricular function have been identified [2, 3]. To date, however, no unifying concept has linked abnormalities in the biochemistry of contraction with the clinical appearance of heart failure. Furthermore, it is not clear whether any given abnormality would be a primary or secondary event.

A structural basis for the appearance of left ventricular dysfunction in the hypertrophied myocardium has also been sought. Both myocyte [4] and nonmyocyte (i.e., intramural coronary vasculature and cardiac interstitium) [5–8] compartments have been considered. Severel promising lines of experimental evidence have implicated the important role for nonmyocyte compartments in the pathologic remodeling of the myocardium. Although definitive correlations with clinical expressions of heart failure remain to be ascertained, the importance of the collagen network and intramyocardial coronary arteries in leading to the failure of this normally efficient muscular pump is now recognized. For example, a remodeling of the existing fibrillar collagen network [9–12], together with a disproportionate accumulation of new collagen, each of which may be termed a reactive fibrosis [10], is responsible for abnormalities in both diastolic and systolic myocardial stiffness [13–17] and subsequent ventricular dysfunction [18–21] of the hypertrophied ventricle.

The structural remodeling of nonmyocyte compartments, however, is not common to the hypertrophic growth of the myocardium in all disease states [8] because hypertrophy is a heterogeneous process. This heterogeneity exists either

---

* This work was supported in part by NHLBI grant no. R05-HL-31701.

because myocyte and nonmyocyte compartments are under the influence of different regulatory mechanisms, or because they respond differently to the same signals. In either case, it is the difference in myocardial structure, promoted by the remodeling of nonmyocyte compartments, which will likely distinguish adaptive from pathologic forms of hypertrophy. In various models of experimental hypertension, having equivalent degrees of left ventricular hypertrophy, the hemodynamic load on the left ventricle would appear to govern myocyte growth. On the other hand, it has been suggested that the remodeling of the collagen network and intramyocardial coronary arteries is based on whether or not the concentration of circulating hormones (e.g., angiotensin II or aldosterone) is increased [20, 22]. Pharmacologic agents, such as the angiotensin converting enzyme inhibitors, which can interfere with such a hormonal response, have shown promise in preventing these detrimental aspects of myocardial remodeling [23, 24].

The purpose of this review is twofold. First, it considers the structural remodeling of the hypertrophied myocardium seen in man with aortic stenosis, coarctation of the aorta, and essential hypertension and in experimental models of aortic constriction and arterial hypertension. The remodeling of the interstitium and intramyocardial coronary arteries by fibrillar collagen is specifically addressed. Second, it considers pharmacologic interventions that may prevent this pathologic aspect of myocardial remodeling in the hypertrophy that accompanies hypertension.

Remodeling of Nonmyocyte Compartments in Hypertrophy

The structural basis for pathologic hypertrophy and heart failure is considered here in man and experimental animals. We focus solely on congenital and acquired aortic valvular stenosis and coarctation of the aorta in man and in the rat and nonhuman primate with either aortic constriction or arterial hypertension.

Structural Basis of Remodeling: The Myocardium as a Three-Compartment Model

In morphologic terms, the myocardium can be viewed as consisting of cardiac myocytes and intramyocardial coronary arteries, arterioles, capillaries, venules, and veins, each of which are contained within a three-dimensional, structural scaffolding consisting of fibrillar type I and III collagens [11, 25, 26]. These muscular, vascular, and collagenous compartments exist in a state of balanced equilibrium that promotes the viability of myocytes and sustains the normal mechanical behavior of the myocardium. A hypertrophic remodeling of the myocardium must preserve this intercompartmental equilibrium if it is to be adaptive (e.g., the hypertrophy of the athlete trained in isometric exercise). Persistent, irreversible intercompartmental disequilibrium constitutes the requisite criteria for pathologic hypertrophy [8].

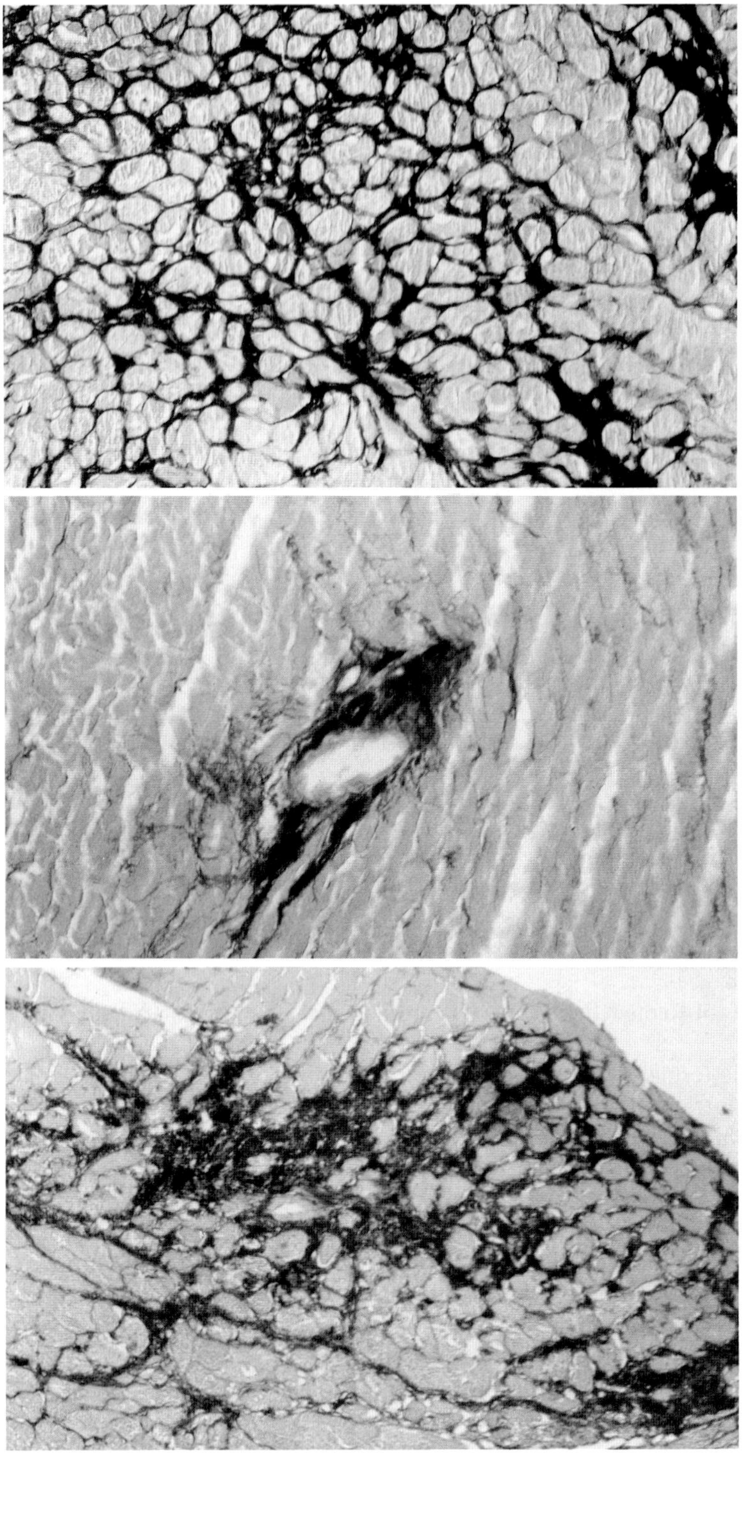

a

b

c

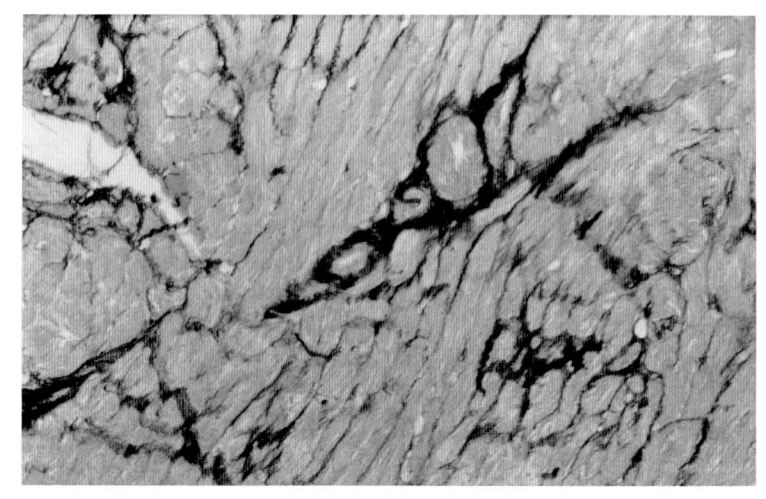

Fig. 1a–d. Patterns of myocardial fibrosis seen in left ventricular hypertrophy. Picrosirius red technique and direct light (×40). Collagen fibers appear *black* and muscle *gray*. **a** A diffuse *interstitial fibrosis* is evident with muscle fibers encircled by fibrillar collagen. **b** The marked accumulation of fibrillar collagen around an intramyocardial coronary artery represents perivascular fibrosis. Septa of collagen radiate outward from their perivascular location into neighboring intermuscular spaces, where they may surround muscle fibers. **c** Microscopic scars, or reparative fibrosis, that have replaced myocytes can be seen together with anchoring collagen fibers that secure the scar to neighboring myocytes. **d** An interstitial and perivascular fibrosis is present together with a microscopic scar in this section of myocardium

Remodeling of the Human Myocardium in Aortic Stenosis, Coarctation of the Aorta, and Arterial Hypertension

An increment in left ventricular myocardial mass (or weight), represented almost entirely by the enlargement of myocytes, is a well-recognized feature of both congenital and acquired aortic valvular stenosis, coarctation of the aorta, and established hypertension. Based on the examination of postmortem tissue, transmural or endomyocardial biopsies of either the right or left ventricle, the portion of myocardium occupied by collagen (i.e., its collagen volume fraction) was found to be increased two- to fourfold in patients with symptomatic heart failure secondary to these conditions [27–33]. This abnormal accumulation of collagen, or fibrosis, is frequently most evident in the endomyocardium, but it is by no means confined solely to this portion of the myocardium.

As shown in Fig. 1, myocardial fibrosis has several different morphologic presentations [12, 34–36]. These include: (a) an interstitial fibrosis (see upper left panel, Fig. 1), that microscopically can give the myocardium a lobulated appearance; (b) a perivascular fibrosis (upper right panel, Fig. 1), involving the adventitia of intramyocardial coronary arteries and from which septa of collagen extend outward between neighboring muscle fibers; (c) a reparative fibrosis (lower left panel, Fig. 1), represented by microscopic scars that replace areas of myocyte loss; and (d) a complex swirling arrangement of collagen fibers, termed a plexiform fibrosis, that is often associated with muscle fiber disarray. Frequently, one or more of these patterns of myocardial fibrosis are seen in the same heart (lower right panel, Fig. 1).

Remodeling of the Myocardium in Experimental Aortic Constriction and Hypertension

An increase in myocardial collagen concentration or its collagen volume fraction has been observed in the left ventricle of the rat after banding the central aorta [37–40], the nonhuman primate [9, 11], and rat [13–15, 18, 41] with experimental hypertension and the rat with genetic hypertension [19, 42, 43]. A similar increase in myocardial collagen concentration has not been found in the rat with chronic anemia [44] or an arteriovenous fistula [45].

In monitoring the remodeling of the fibrillar collagen network over time, a number of laboratories [13–15, 20, 24, 46] have found that both the interstitial and perivascular fibrosis are progressive in nature. The interrelationship between the septa of collagen that radiate from intramural vessels, to create a streaky appearance to the myocardium, and the accumulation of fibrillar collagen between muscle fibers and muscle bundles, or the interstitial fibrosis, is unclear. Nevertheless, these reactive (nonreparative) patterns of fibrosis are composed of heavy perimysial and endomysial collagen fibers [9, 12, 13], consisting primarily of type I collagen [47]. These fibers, respectively, encircle groups of muscle fibers, or muscle bundles, and individual muscle fibers. The increased dimension of the peri- and endomysium of the collagen network resembles the collagen network seen in slow-twitch skeletal muscle (vis à vis fast-twitch muscle, where these components are less well developed) [48].

In later phases of established hypertrophy seen with renovascular hypertension [20, 21] and genetic hypertension [42], myocardial fibrosis is particularly evident in the endomyocardium. A reparative (or replacement) fibrosis, which occupies the space created by myocyte loss, may also be evident at this juncture [11, 12, 20]. Based on the initial alignment of thick and thin collagen fibers, it has been proposed that the reactive and reparative forms of myocardial fibrosis can be distinguished from one another [12, 16, 49].

Functional Consequences of Collagen Network Remodeling

Type I collagen fibers have a tensile strength greater than steel [50, 51]. The majority (i.e., 85%) of the total collagen protein pool in the myocardium consists of type I collagen [11]. Type III collagen, which is more distensible, represents 11% of this pool, while type IV (membranous) and type V (pericellular) collagens are found in lesser quantities. It is not necessary for the concentration of type I collagen to increase very much in order for myocardial stiffness to be altered significantly. In deriving structure-function correlates, it is equally informative to consider the location (e.g., in-series versus in parallel), configuration (e.g., wavy, taut, corkscrew), an alignment of collagen fibers with respect to myocytes [10, 14,

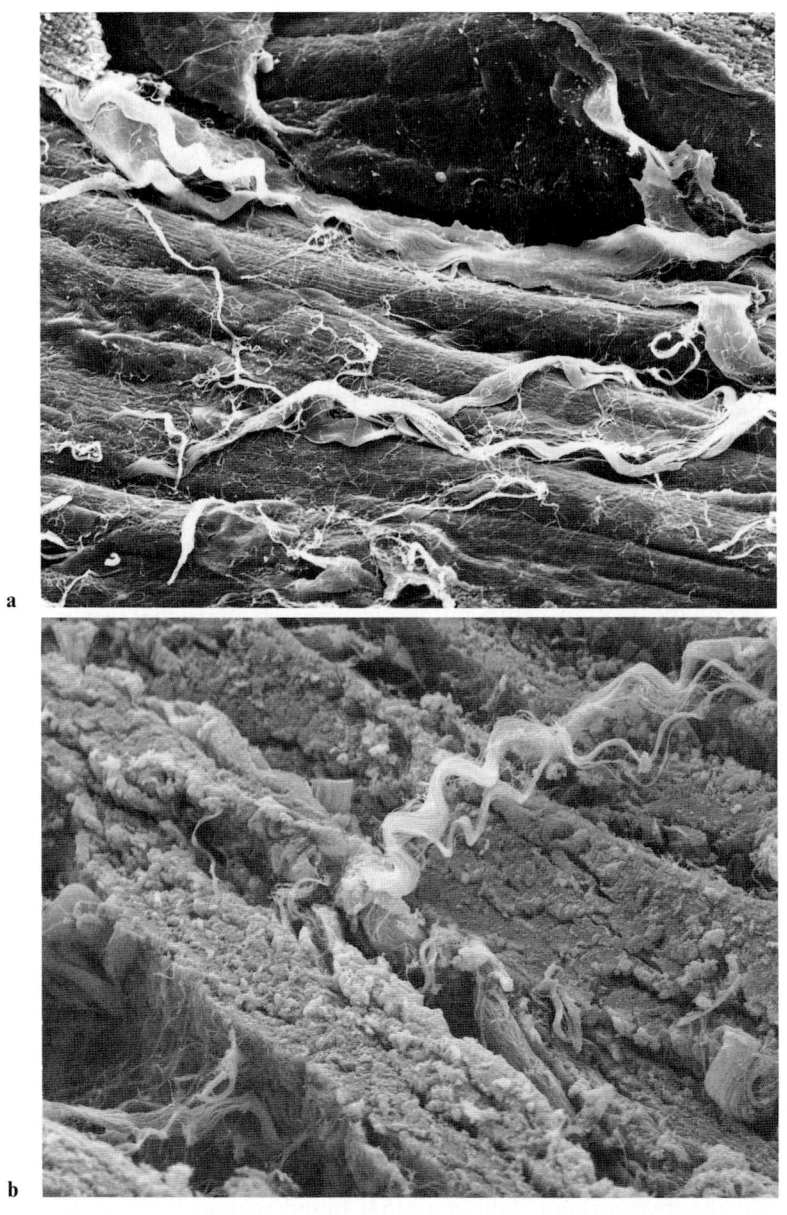

Fig. 2a, b. Scanning electron microscopy of perimysial collagen fibers found in the normal myocardium. **a** Wavy configuration ($\times 700$). **b** Corkscrew configuration ($\times 1500$)

16]. Figure 2 demonstrates the wavy and corkscrew configurations of perimysial collagen fibers that exist in the myocardium. In the upper left panel of Fig. 1, the in parallel arrangement of collagen and muscle, represented by the interstitial fibrosis, is seen while in the lower left panel the reparative fibrosis represents an inseries addition of collagen relative to muscle fibers.

Systolic and Diastolic Myocardial Stiffness

The stiffness of the intact myocardium can be assessed from it's stress-strain relation [52]. Stress is derived for the thick-walled myocardium from the product of ventricular chamber pressure and cross-sectional chamber area divided by the cross-sectional area of myocardium. The stress calculation normalizes for differences in ventricular chamber size and myocardial mass between different hearts. Strain is derived for a circumferential fiber length, located in the midwall of the ventricle, normalized to its unstretched length at zero filling pressure.

The slope of the linear, developed systolic stress-strain relation obtained in the isovolumetrically beating ventricle over the filling pressure range of 0–25 mmHg, provides an estimate of active stiffness. The end-diastolic stress-strain relation is normally only slightly curvilinear over the physiologic range of filling pressures. With fibrosis, this relation becomes more curvilinear, and therefore the slope of this relation, representing passive stiffness, is given for a particular strain (e.g., 5% or 10%).

Studies by Doering et al. [13] and Jalil et al. [14, 15] indicate that during the early established and established phases of hypertrophy, when there is an interstitial fibrosis throughout the myocardium and a two- to threefold increase in collagen volume fraction, active stiffness is increased above that seen in the normal left ventricle. Passive stiffness is also increased, but only for higher strains. This implies that left ventricular systolic and diastolic function are preserved for normal filling volumes; at larger filling volumes, however, such as those seen with the heightened venous return of isotonic exercise or with volume expansion, diastolic stiffness is abnormal and would lead to an excessive elevation in left ventricular filling pressure. McElroy et al. [53] have found that pulmonary occlusive wedge pressure, which was normal at rest, may rise abnormally during incremental treadmill exercise and be associated with a fall in stroke volume, in patients with hypertension and minimal electrocardiographic evidence of left ventricular hypertrophy. Averill et al. [18] and Pfeffer et al. [19] reported that the left ventricular function curve, or rise in stroke volume for increments in filling pressure of the left ventricle in response to volume loading, is impaired in rats with renovascular or genetic hypertension, respectively.

During the late phase of established hypertrophy, as the disproportionate endomyocardial fibrosis becomes quite evident, a marked rise in diastolic stiffness is seen at all strains while active stiffness now declines [14]. The reparative component of the endomyocardial fibrosis is associated with a meshwork of collagen fibers that surround adjacent myocytes, and which serve to anchor these scars into the myocardium. Jalil et al. [54] found that with the appearance of these anchoring fibers and the reduction in length-dependent force generation a progressive atrophy of these viable myocytes, now encircled by collagen, would ensue. This serves to explain the commonly observed variation in myocyte size found in the endomyocardium with late established hypertrophy. Capasso et al. [21] have shown that late in established hypertrophy, with the marked fibrosis of the entire myocardium, including 25% of the endomyocardium which is now occupied by fibrous tissue, abnormalities in diastolic and systolic left ventricular function are present.

Prevention of Collagen Network Remodeling in Hypertrophy

The ideal pharmacologic approach to preventing pathologic hypertrophy due to myocardial fibrosis would be based on understanding pathogenetic mechanisms involved in enhancing collagen synthesis and/or cardiac fibroblast proliferation. Cardiac fibroblasts, not myocytes, contain the messenger RNA for type I and III collagens [55, 56]. Much work needs to be done in this area before definitive recommendations can be made. However, several promising reports have appeared dealing with the prevention of myocardial fibrosis in the rat with experimental or genetic (SHR) hypertension.

Prevention of Myocardial Fibrosis in Experimental Hypertension

Wiener and coworkers [57–60] have shown that the permeability of intramyocardial coronary arteries is increased in rats with 1–4 weeks of renovascular hypertension (RHT) and have suggested that this is the result of alterations in interendothelial cell integrity. His laboratory also noted that the morphologic remodeling of the coronary vasculature in RHT was similar to that seen within hours of an angiotensin infusion. Engler et al. [61] have demonstrated angiotensin-induced abnormalities of the coronary endothelial cell membrane which was followed by cardiac fibroblast proliferation that began within the media and adventitia of small intramural arteries and arterioles. Complementary to these morphologic studies, Laine [62] observed that cardiac lymph flow and coronary microvascular permeability were each increased in the dog with RHT for 4 weeks. Collectively, these findings suggest that angiotensin is responsible for initiating the events that led to perivascular and interstitial fibrosis in RHT. Accordingly, Jalil et al. [23] pretreated rats with the angiotensin converting enzyme inhibitor captopril prior to creating RHT. After 8 weeks of RHT and captopril therapy, these patterns of fibrosis were not seen, and the expected abnormal elevation in diastolic stiffness was absent. Michel and coworkers [24, 63] have suggested that another angiotensin converting enzyme inhibitor, perindopril, is also effective in preventing myocardial fibrosis, as well as the fibrinoid necrosis and fibrous endarteritis of afferent arterioles and interlobar and arcuate arteries of the nonischemic kidney of the rat with RHT. This vasculoprotective effect of perindopril was not seen in rats with RHT that received a combination of clonidine, hydralazine, and furosemide.

In rats with arterial hypertension secondary to the chronic administration of deoxycorticosterone, Ooshima et al. [64] observed that collagen synthesis in the myocardium and aorta was enhanced, and that this could be reduced to control levels with the catecholamine-depleting agent reserpine. This was not the case for the diuretic hydrochlorothiazide and suggests that hormonal factors, like the catecholamines, may be involved in mediating myocardial fibrosis in this model of hypertension; it further suggests that hemodynamic factors are less important.

Prevention of Myocardial Fibrosis in Spontaneous Hypertensive Rats (SHR)

Sen and Bumpus [43] found that even prior to their becoming hypertensive myocardial collagen synthesis was increased in 4-week-old rats with genetic hypertension. Later, with established hypertension and hypertrophy, collagen synthesis was once again increased. The mechanisms responsible for these elevations in collagen synthesis are unclear, but would account for the increase in myocardial collagen concentration seen in adult SHR. Various antihypertensive agents, given alone or in combination, were able to prevent the late increase in collagen synthesis [43] while captopril treatment, initiated at 3 weeks of age, prevented the subsequent increase in collagen concentration [65].

Once hypertrophy is established and myocardial collagen volume fraction is increased in SHR, the regression of hypertrophy with short-term (6 weeks) antihypertensive therapy has been associated with an increase in collagen concentration [41, 66, 67]. Motz and Strauer [68] recently found that long-term (20 weeks) treatment with the calcium channel blocker nifedipine reduced collagen volume fraction together with a regression in myocardial mass. Whether this represents a specific benefit of nifedipine or the longer duration of treatment is uncertain.

In summary, several promising lines of medical therapy may prove effective in preventing the fibrosis and pathologic hypertrophy which accompanies the remodeling of the myocardium in systemic hypertension. Such pharmacologic agents would thereby alleviate the appearance of ventricular dysfunction and symptomatic heart failure.

References

1. Kannel WB (1989) Epidemiological aspects of heart failure. In: Weber KT (ed) Congestive heart failure. Cardiol Clin 7:1–9
2. Wikman-Coffelt J, Parmley WW, Mason DT (1979) The cardiac hypertrophy process. Analyses of factors determining pathological vs. physiological development. Circ Res 45:697–707
3. Schwart A, Sordahl LA, Entman ML, Allen JC, Reddy YS, Goldstein MA, Luchi RJ, Wyborny LE (1973) Abnormal biochemistry in myocardial failure. Am J Cardiol 32:407–422
4. Maron BJ, Ferraus VJ, Roberts WC (1975) Ultrastructural features of degenerated cardiac muscle cells in patients with cardiac hypertrophy. Am J Pathol 79:387–396
5. Anversa P, Ricci R, Olivetti G (1986) Quantitative structural analysis of the myocardium during physiologic growth and induced cardiac hypertrophy: a review. J Am Coll Cardiol 7:1140–1149
6. Tomanek RJ, Palmer PJ, Pfeiffer GL, Schreiber KL, Eastham CL, Marcus ML (1986) Morphometry of canine coronary arteries, arterioles, and capillaries during hypertension and left ventricular hypertrophy. Circ Res 58:38–46
7. Rakusan K, Wicker P, Abdul-Samad M, Healy B, Turek Z (1987) Failure of swimming exercise to improve capillarization in cardiac hypertrophy of renal hypertensive rats. Circ Res 61:641–647
8. Weber KT, Clark WA, Janicki JS, Shroff SG (1987) Physiologic versus pathologic hypertrophy and the pressure-overload myocardium. J Cardiovasc Pharmacol 10:537–549
9. Abrahams C, Janicki JS, Weber KT (1987) Myocardial hypertrophy in *Macaca fascicularis*: structural remodeling of the collagen matrix. Lab Invest 56:676–683

10. Weber KT, Janicki JS, Shroff SG, Pick R, Abrahams C, Chen RM, Bashey RI (1988) Collagen compartment remodeling in the pressure overloaded left ventricle. J Appl Cardiol 3:37–46
11. Weber KT, Janicki JS, Shroff SG, Pick R, Chen RM, Bashey RI (1988) Collagen remodeling of the pressure overloaded, hypertrophied nonhuman primate myocardium. Circ Res 62:757–765
12. Pick R, JE, Janicki JS, Weber KT (1989) Myocardial fibrosis in nonhuman primate with pressure overload hypertrophy. Am J Pathol 135:771–781
13. Doering CW, Jalil JE, Janicki JS, Pick R, Aghili S, Abrahams C, Weber KT (1988) Collagen network remodeling and diastolic stiffness of the rat left ventricle with pressure overload hypertrophy. Cardiovasc Res 22:686–695
14. Jalil JE, Doering CW, Janicki JS, Pick R, Shroff S, Weber KT (1989) Fibrillar collagen and myocardial stiffness in the intact hypertrophied rat left ventricle. Circ Res 64:1041–1050
15. Jalil JE, Doering CW, Janicki JS, Pick R, Clark WA, Weber KT (1988) Structural vs contractile protein remodeling and myocardial stiffness in hypertrophied rat left ventricle. J Mol Cell Cardiol 20:1179–1187
16. Carroll EP, Janicki JS, Pick R, Weber KT (1989) Myocardial stiffness and reparative fibrosis following coronary embolization in the rat. Cardiovasc Res 23:657–670
17. Bing OHL, Fanburg BL, Brooks WW, Matsushita S (1978) The effect of the lathyrogen β-amino proprionitrile (BAPN) on the mechanical properties of experimentally hypertrophied rat cardiac muscle. Circ Res 43:632–637
18. Averill DB, Ferrario CM, Tarazi RC, Sen S, Bajbus R (1976) Cardiac performance in rats with renal hypertension. Circ Res 38:280–288
19. Pfeffer JM, Pfeffer MA, Fishbein MC, Froehlich ED (1979) Cardiac function and morphology with aging in the spontaneously hypertensive rat. Am J Physiol 6:H461–H468
20. Weber KT, Janicki JS, Pick R, Capasso J, Anversa P (1990) Myocardial fibrosis and pathologic hypertrophy in the rat with renovascular hypertension. Am J Cardiol 65:(in press)
21. Capasso JM, Palackal T, Olivetti G, Anversa P (1990) Left ventricular failure induced by long term hypertension in rats. Circ Res (in press)
22. Weber KT, Janicki JS (1989) Angiotensin II and myocardial remodeling. Br J Clin Pharmacol 28:1415–1505
23. Jalil JE, Janicki JS, Shroff SG, Pick R, Weber KT (1989) Captopril pretreatment and myocardial fibrosis and stiffness in renovascular hypertensive rats. J Am Coll Cardiol 13:82A (abstr)
24. Michel JB, Salzmann JL, De Lourdes Cerol M, Dussaule JC, Azizi M, Corman B, Camilleri JP, Corvol P (1988) Myocardial effect of converting enzyme inhibition in hypertensive and normotensive rats. Am J Med [Suppl 3A]:12–21
25. Medugorac I, Jacob R (1983) Characterization of left ventricular collagen in the rat. Cardiovasc Res 17:15–21
26. Dawson R, Milne G, Williams RB (1982) Changes in the collagen of rat heart in Cooper-deficiency-induced cardiac hypertrophy. Cardiovasc Res 16:559–565
27. Schwarz F, Flameng W, Schaper J, Hehrlein F (1978) Correlation between myocardial strcuture and diastolic properties of the heart in chronic aortic valve disease: effects of corrective surgery. Am J Cardiol 42:895–903
28. Caspari PG, Newcomb M, Gibson K, Harris P (1977) Collagen in the normal and hypertrophied human ventricle. Cardiovasc Res 11:554–558
29. Hess OM, Schneider J, Koch R, Bamert C, Grimm J, Krayenbuehl HP (1981) Diastolic function and myocardial structure in patients with myocardial hypertrophy. Sepcial reference to normalized viscoelastic data. Circulation 63:360–371
30. Schaper J, Schaper W (1983) Ultrastructural correlates of reduced cardiac function in human heart disease. Eur Heart J 4 [Suppl A]:35–42
31. Oldershaw PJ, Brooksby IAB, Davies MJ, Coltart DJ, Jenkins BS, Webb-Peploe MM (1980) Correlations of fibrosis in endomyocardial biopsies from patients with aortic valve disease. Br Heart J 44:609–611
32. Krayenbuehl HP, Hess OM, Monrad ES, Schneider J, Mall G, Turina M (1989) Left ventricular myocardial structure in aortic valve disease before, intermediate, and late after aortic valve replacement. Circulation 79:744–755

33. Pearlman ES, Weber KT, Janicki JS, Pietra G, Fishman AP (1982) Muscle fiber orientation and connective tissue content in the hypertrophied human heart. Lab Invest 46:158–164
34. Anderson KR, St. John Sutton MG, Lie JT (1979) Histopathological types of cardiac fibrosis in myocardial disease. J Pathol 128:79–85
35. Naeye RL, Liedtke AJ (1976) Consequences of intramyocardial arterial lesions in aortic valvular stenosis. Am J Pathol 85:569–580
36. Tanaka M, Fujiwara H, Onodera T, Wu D, Matsuda M, Hamashime Y, Kawai C (1987) Quantitative analysis of narrowing of intramyocardial small arteries in normal hearts, hypertensive hearts, and hearts with hypertrophic cardiomyopathy. Circulation 75:1130–1139
37. Grove D, Zak R, Nair KG, Aschenbrenner V (1969) Biochemical correlates of cardiac hypertrophy. IV. Observations on the cellular organization of growth during myocardial hypertrophy in the rat. Circ Res 25:473–485
38. Skosey JL, Zak R, Martin AF (1972) Biochemical correlates of cardiac hypertrophy. V. Labeling of collagen, myosin and nuclear DNA experimental myocardial hypertrophy in the rat. Circ Res 31:145–157
39. Cutilletta AF, Dowell RT, Rudnik M, Arcilla RA, Zak R (1975) Regression of myocardial hypertrophy: experimental model, changes in heart weight, nucleic acids and collagen. J Mol Cell Cardiol 7:767–781
40. Bing OHL, Matsushita S, Fanburg BL, Levine HJ (1971) Mechanical properties of rat cardiac muscle during experimental hypertrophy. Circ Res 28:233–245
41. Sen S, Tarazi RC, Bumpus FM (1981) Reversal of cardiac hypertrophy in renal hypertensive rats: medical vs. surgical therapy. Am J Physiol 240:H408–H412
42. Pfeffer MA, Pfeffer JM, Froehlich ED (1976) Pumping ability of the hypertrophying left ventricle of the spontaneously hypertensive rat. Circ Res 38:423–429
43. Sen S, Bumpus FM (1979) Collagen synthesis in development and reversal of cardiac hypertrophy in spontaneously hypertensive rats. Am J Cardiol 44:954–958
44. Bartosova D, Chvapil M, Korecky B, Poupa O, Rakusan K, Turek Z, Vizek M (1969) The growth of the muscular and collagenous parts of the rat heart in various forms of cardiomegaly. J Physiol 200:185–195
45. Michel JB, Salzmann JL, Ossondo Nlom M, Bruneval P, Barres D, Camilleri JP (1986) Morphometric analysis of collagen network and plasma perfused capillary bed in the myocardium of rats during evolution of cardiac hypertrophy. Basic Res Cardiol 81:142–154
46. Thiedemann KU, Holubarsch C, Medugorac I, Jacob R (1983) Connective tissue content and myocardial stiffness in pressure overload hypertrophy. A combined study of morphologic, morphometric, biochemical and mechanical parameters. Basic Res Cardiol 78:140–155
47. Chapman D, Weber KT, Eghbali M (1989) Accumulation and localization of types I and III collagen in the hypertrophied rat left ventricle FASEB 3:A621 (abstr)
48. Rowe RWD (1974) Collagen fiber arrangement in intramuscular connective tissue. Changes associated with muscle shortening and their possible relevance to raw meat toughness measurements. J Food Technol 9:501–508
49. Pick R, Jalil JE, Janicki JS, Weber KT (1954) The fibrillar nature and structure of isoproterenol-induced myocardial fibrosis in the rat. Am J Pathol 134:365–371
50. Burton AC (1954) Relation of structure to function of the tissues of the wall of blood vessels. Physiol Rev 34:619–642
51. Parry DAD, Craig AS (1988) Collagen fibrils during development and maturation and their contribution to the mechanical attributes of connective tissue. In: Nimni ME (ed) Collagen, Vol 2. CRC, Boca Raton, pp 1–23
52. Weber KT, Janicki JS, Hunter WC, Shroff SG, Pearlman ES, Fishman AP (1982) The contractile behavior of the heart and its functional coupling to the circulation. Prog Cardiovasc Dis 24:375–400
53. McElroy PA, Janicki JS, Weber KT (1988) Early ventricular dysfunction in hypertensive patients with preserved aerobic capacity. J Am Coll Cardiol 11:142A (abstr.)
54. Jalil JE, Janicki JS, Pick R, Abrahams C, Weber KT (1989) Fibrosis-induced reduction of endomyocardium in the rat following isoproterenol. Circ Res 65:258–264

55. Eghbali M, Czaja MJ, Zeyel M, Weiner FR, Zern MA, Seifter S, Blumenfeld OO (1988) Collagen chain mRNAs in isolated heart cells from young and adult rats. J Mol Cell Cardiol 20:267–276
56. Eghbali M, Blumenfeld OO, Seifter S, Buttrick PM, Leinwand LA, Robinson TF, Zern MA, Giambrone MA (1989) Localization of types I, III, and IV collagen mRNAs in rat heart cells by in situ hybridization. J Mol Cell Cardiol 21:103–113
57. Wiener J, Giacomelli F (1973) The cellular pathology of experimental hypertension. VII. Structure and permeability of the mesenteric vasculature in angiotensin-induced hypertension. Am J Pathol 72:221–240
58. Wiener J, Lattes RG, Meltzer BG, Spiro D (1969) The cellular pathology of experimental hypertension. IV. Evidence for increased vascular permeability. Am J Pathol 54:187–207
59. Bhan RD, Giacomelli F, Wiener J (1978) Ultrastructure of coronary arteries and myocardium in experimental hypertension. Exp Mol Pathol 29:66–81
60. Giacomelli F, Anversa P, Wiener J (1976) Effect of angiotensin-induced hypertension on rat coronary arteries and myocardium. Am J Pathol 84:111–125
61. Engler E, Matthias D, Becker CH (1980) Pathomorphological reactions of myocardium and intramural vessels of rats in the course of hypertension induced by depot angiotensin. Autoradiographic, light and electron microscopic investigations. Exp Pathol 18:37–51
62. Laine GA (1988) Microvascular changes in the heart during chronic arterial hypertension. Circ Res 62:953–960
63. Michel JB, Dussaule JC, Choudat L, Auzan C, Nochy D, Corvol P, Menard J (1986) Effects of antihypertensive treatment in one-clip, two kidney hypertension in rats. Kidney Int 29:1011–1020
64. Ooshima A, Fuller GC, Cardinale GJ, Spector S, Udenfriend S (1974) Increased collagen synthesis in blood vessels of hypertensive rats and its reversal by antihypertensive agents. Proc Natl Acad Sci USA 71:3019–3023
65. Sen S, Tarazi RC, Bumpus FM (1980) Effect of converting enzyme inhibitor (SQ14,225) on myocardial hypertrophy in spontaneously hypertensive rats. Hypertension 2:169–176
66. Sen S, Tarazi RC, Bumpus FM (1976) Biochemical changes associated with development and reversal of cardiac hypertrophy in spontaneously hypertensive rats. Cardiovasc Res 10:254–261
67. Sen S, Tarazi RC, Bumpus FM (1977) Cardiac hypertrophy and antihypertensive therapy. Cardiovasc Res 11:427–433
68. Motz W, Strauer BE (1989) Left ventricular function and collagen content after regression of hypertensive hypertrophy. Hypertension 13:43–50

Treatment of Heart Failure by "Afterload" Reduction: Vasodilator or Angiotensin Converting Enzyme Inhibitor?

P. A. Poole-Wilson

Introduction

The objectives of treatment in chronic heart failure are prevention, relief of symptoms, retardation of the disease process, and reduction of mortality. The traditional therapy is with diuretics and digoxin, the use and dose of individual drugs being guided largely by physical signs and symptoms. In the last two decades the concept of "vasodilatation" has emerged, and vasodilators have become widely used for treatment, prevention and to alter mortality [1–3].

The term vasodilator is used loosely to include any drug which brings about relaxation of the arteries and veins. Thus the word can refer to direct-acting agents such as nitrates and hydralazine, receptor-dependent drugs such as prazosin, calcium antagonists and the angiotensin converting enzyme (ACE) inhibitors. The terminology implies that the efficacy of these drugs in heart failure is entirely dependent on their ability to relax smooth muscle. In this chapter I argue that all vasodilators do not have similar effects, that most vasodilators are not particularly advantageous in heart failure, and that the ACE inhibitors may exert their more beneficial effects by mechanisms relatively specific to that group of drugs. The ACE inhibitors should not be grouped with other vasodilators.

Syndromes of Heart Failure

Heart failure covers many clinical conditions, such as acute heart failure, circulatory collapse and chronic heart failure (Table 1). By chronic heart failure is meant a chronic clinical syndrome caused by an abnormality of the heart and recognised

Table 1. A simple classification of terms used to describe syndromes of heart failure

Entity	Synonym or variant
Acute heart failure	Pulmonary oedema
Circulatory collapse	"Shock" (poor peripheral perfusion, oliguria hypotension)
Chronic heart failure	Untreated, congestive, undulating; treated, compensated

Redundant terms: right, left, forward, backward, high and low output.

by a characteristic pattern of haemodynamic, renal, neural and hormonal responses [4, 5]. When treated, the clinical signs of heart failure may be few. The natural history of chronic heart failure is unsufficiently studied, but many physicians recognise a pattern where patients are regularly readmitted with what appears to be undulating heart failure. The cause of the intermittent periods of deterioration may be evident, for example, an arrhythmia or infection, or it may be unknown.

An important distinction must be made between heart failure and ventricular dysfunction. Ventricular dysfunction is the consequence of damage to the myocardium when the patient is maintained in a steady state without the need for any drug treatment. Such patients may be limited in the ability to exercise. Heart failure exists when ventricular dysfunction coexists with evidence of a substantial body response, particularly the retention of sodium and water, and a diuretic is prescribed.

Current Treatment

A scheme for the treatment of heart failure is shown in Table 2. Digoxin is used in atrial fibrillation to control heart rate, but controversy continues over the use of digoxin in sinus rhythm [6, 7]. In part this controversy reflects the lack of data to answer relevant clinical questions and in part the natural reluctance of medical practitioners to change traditional therapeutic practice.

The three key questions currently facing the cardiologist in the treatment of heart failure are (a) what drug(s) to use as initial therapy, (b) what drug to add (or to increase the dose of existing drugs) if symptoms persist, and (c) whether other drugs should be prescribed early in the belief that they alter the natural history of the disease.

Recent work [8] has shown that the body fluid compartments (plasma volume, extracellular volume, total body sodium) are normal in patients who have been

Table 2. A scheme for the treatment of chronic heart failure

General	No added salt	Treat hypertension
	Maintain optimal weight	Detect alcohol abuse
	Stop smoking	Prevent coronary disease
Mild	Thiazide diuretic	ACE inhibitor?
	Digoxin if in atrial fibrillation	
	Potassium therapy	
Moderate	Loop diuretic	Potassium therapy?
	ACE inhibitor	
Severe	Increase loop diuretic	Nitrates
	Mix diuretics	Inotropic drug?
	Metolazone	Digoxin?
	ACE inhibitor	Spironolactone?

treated with diuretics, and in whom the physician on the basis of simple clinical observations but including the chest X ray and blood electrolytes is of the opinion that the patient is receiving an adequate dose of diuretic. There is no logic therefore in increasing the dose of diuretic in such patients.

Vasodilators

The concept that patients with heart failure would benefit from vasodilatation was born two decades ago [1-3]. The objective was to improve symptoms, delay the progression of damage to the heart muscle and to alter mortality. The reasons for advocating such therapy were the finding that the systemic resistance was greatly increased in heart failure and the observation that vasodilators such as nitrates increased cardiac output and reduced left ventricular filling pressure (Fig. 1). These two haemodynamic variables were thought to relate to the two major symptoms of chronic heart failure, namely fatigue and shortness of breath.

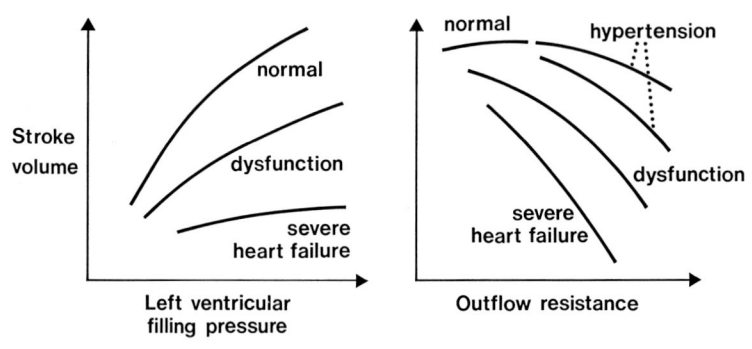

Fig. 1. The haemodynamic mechanism by which vasodilators decrease left ventricular end-diastolic pressure but increase cardiac output in heart failure. Note that the relation between cardiac output and filling pressure is flat in heart failure whilst the relation to "afterload" is steep

Cause of Heart Failure and Relevance to Treatment

Physicians at present distinguish between heart failure due to the manifestations of atheromatous coronary artery disease and that due to cardiomyopathy. The cardiomyopathies are divided into dilated, restrictive and hypertrophic on clinical criteria. This distinction rests largely on the presence or not of atheroma in the coronary arteries. The classification overlooks the importance of shape, cell slippage, hypertrophy, cell orientation, incoordinate contraction, fibrosis and numerous other variables [9]. The response of the heart to exercise differs if heart failure is due to ischaemia or a cardiomyopathy. Little information is available on the response to vasodilators when heart failure is due to different types of cardiac abnormality. There are likely to be selected subgroups who respond particularly favourably to nitrates, beta antagonists, inotropic drugs, vasodilators or ACE inhibitors.

A popular concept is to distinguish between heart failure due to systolic function and diastolic abnormalities [10–13]. This is a very old idea [14] and is of obvious importance in hypertrophic cardiomyopathy, hypertension, following aortic valve surgery and the small fibrotic heart in the presence of a tachycardia. Evidence for a fundamentally different approach to the treatment of diastolic heart failure is not available although theoretical reasons can be put forward for the use of particular groups of drugs such as the calcium antagonists or beta blockers.

Progression of Heart Failure and Natural History

The prognosis of heart failure is poor, varying from a mortality of 50% per annum in severe heart failure [15, 16] to one of 25% per annum if all patients with heart failure are included [17]. About 15% of patients have a good prognosis, surviving for up to 20 years [17]. These may be patients in whom either the original diagnosis was wrong, or who had a temporary abnormality of cardiac function from which a full recovery was possible.

The nature of the progression of heart failure is unclear. Two popular concepts are shown in Fig. 2. In one the increase in the response in the body to the greater peripheral resistance is believed to impose an increased workload on the ventricular muscle and thus to exacerbate damage to the cardiac muscle. Evidence for this hypothesis comes from a rat model of heart failure in which a coronary artery is occluded [18]. Progressive enlargement of the ventricle occurs in those animals that develop failure, and benefit accrues from treatment with ACE inhibitors. In two studies ACE inhibitors have been introduced soon after acute myocardial infarction in man. In one [19] the results were essentially negative, and in the other [20] a small benefit was detected in that the enlargement of the ventricle was slightly reduced by an ACE inhibitor. The mechanism by which the muscle is progressively damaged due to increased wall stress is uncertain but could be due to ischaemia, hypertrophy, fibrosis, or a shape change in the ventricle.

Fig. 2. Two mechanisms for the progression of heart failure. *Left*, an increase of wall stress due to systemic vasoconstriction causes damage to the myocardium. *Right*, fluid retention is the cause of worsening heart failure

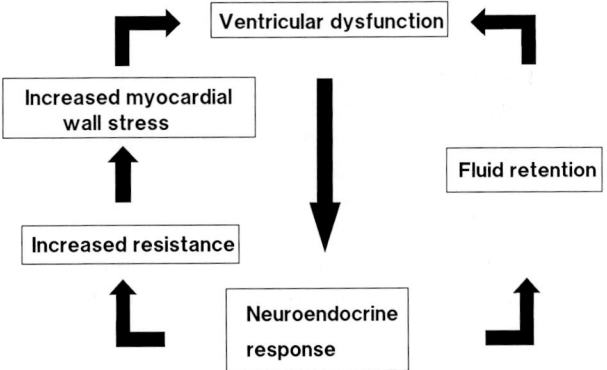

The second scheme (Fig. 2) is that the body's response to heart failure results in activation of numerous neural and hormonal systems resulting in greater retention of salt and water by the kidney. This spontaneous tendency could account for "undulating" heart failure.

A third possibility is that the progression of damage to the myocardium is determined more by the nature of the initiating disease, for example, coronary artery disease or intake of alcohol, rather than a direct consequence of the heart failure itself. According to this idea progression of coronary artery disease and further coronary events would be the major reason for worsening heart failure in many patients with myocardial ischaemia as the cause of heart failure.

Causes of Death from Heart Failure. The cause of death in heart failure is also a contentious issue. In one sense, of little importance, all patients with heart failure die of an arrhythmia. Arrhythmias are common in patients with heart failure [21], and numerous publications have claimed that sudden death occurs in as many as 50% of patients. The implication would be that anti-arrhythmic therapy would be advantageous. The argument rests on whether the arrhythmia occurring at the time of death is an opportunistic arrhythmia or associated with a change in the severity of heart failure. In the CONSENSUS study [15] the improvement in longevity was due almost entirely to delayed progression of heart failure either because of altered afterload on the heart or a reduction of the retention of salt and water (Fig. 2). The third cause of death to consider is a coronary event or sudden exacerbation of the original cause of heart failure.

The difficulty with ascribing 50% of deaths to opportunistic arrhythmias and classifying such deaths as sudden death is the definition of sudden death. Sometimes this is defined as death within 6 h of the patient having been seen alive and well. Even if the time limit is reduced to 1 h, that is still plenty of time for the patient to have a myocardial infarction, a period of myocardial ischaemia or the onset of pulmonary oedema in association with a transient fall of cardiac function. The issue will be resolved only if trials with drugs known to have an effect only on the occurrence of arrhythmias are used in heart failure and shown to reduce mortality. Initial studies are not encouraging.

Symptoms, Peripheral Vascular Resistance, and Skeletal Muscle Blood Flow

Recent work has cast doubt on the simple idea that shortness of breath and fatigue are directly related to the left ventricular end-diastolic pressure and cardiac output in patients with chronic heart failure treated with diuretics. Undoubtedly in acute heart failure shortness of breath is linked rather directly to the left ventricular end-diastolic pressure, and interventions which lower that pressure bring rapid relief to the patient. In patients with severe chronic heart failure treated adequately with diuretics so that sodium and water overload are absent the evidence suggests that this simple relation does not exist [22]. Within a group of patients with severe heart failure there is no relation between the left ventricular end-diastolic pressure and exercise capacity assessed as the maximal oxygen consumption [23, 24]. If end-diastolic pressure were a major determinant of exercise capacity, it would be expected that exercise would terminate at a given high pressure. Different types of exercise test are associated with different symptoms [23]. For example, a fast exercise test terminates with shortness of breath and a slow exercise test with fatigue, but the end-diastolic pressure at the end of the two types of exercise are the same. Drugs, particularly vasodilators, alter the end-diastolic pressure at the end of exercise but given acutely to patients with heart failure do not increase exercise capacity [25–27]. These three lines of evidence indicate that the filling pressure of the ventricle is not a key determinant of exercise performance in patients with chronic heart failure treated with diuretics.

The cardiac output is reduced in patients in chronic heart failure both at rest and on exercise. The redistribution of blood flow is such that the blood flow to the brain and heart is relatively well preserved whilst flow to skin, the splanchnic circulation and the kidney is selectively reduced [28, 29]. The effects of most vasodilators appear not to be selective so that the increased cardiac output due to the fall in wall tension in the heart consequent on arteriolar vasodilatation is directed to the skin and splanchnic circulation and not to exercising skeletal muscle.

An important new principle is emerging, namely that unless blood flow to exercising skeletal muscle is increased during treatment of heart failure (when sodium and water retention has already been eliminated with diuretics) exercise capacity will not increase. The point is almost self-evident. The ability of normal persons or those with heart disease is severely limited in the absence of blood flow to skeletal muscle. The amount of exercise which can be achieved anaerobically is small, and alteration of this amount will not have a great effect on the symptoms of patients. At peak exercise in chronic heart failure the femoral venous oxygen content is almost zero, blood pressure is not greatly reduced, and blood flow is about one-fifth of normal [30]. The vascular resistance must therefore be increased five-fold. This resistance is independent of the cardiac output. Unless the resistance is reduced by therapy, blood flow cannot increase, and a drug is unlikely to be beneficial.

Two studies [31, 32] have shown clearly that the increase of exercise capacity associated with ACE inhibitors is related to the increased blood flow to skeletal muscle. This effect may not be the only mechanism for the improvement in the patient's condition but certainly seems to be a major factor.

The cause of the increased resistance in the vascular bed of exercising muscle is not known (Table 3). Certainly it is not caused solely by vasoconstriction due to activation of the sympathetic system or the renin-angiotensin system since inhibitors of these two systems have no acute effect on exercising capacity and only a limited effect on resistance. The benefit from ACE inhibitors is apparent over a period of approximately 4 weeks [33]. Other possible mechanisms for the increased resistance include abnormal endothelial cell function, cell oedema, compression from adjacent oedematous tissues, vasoconstriction of smooth muscle and a reduction in the capillary density. Studies of skeletal muscle from patients with heart failure [34–36] have shown a wide variety of abnormalities such as muscle atrophy, lipid accumulation, reduction of type 2B fibres but normal capillary distribution. Muscle function and biochemistry are also abnormal [37, 38].

Table 3. Causes of increased peripheral resistance in the exercising skeletal muscle of patients with chronic heart failure

1. Tissue oedema
2. Endothelial cell oedema
3. Arteriolar constriction
   – Sodium/calcium exchange
   – Unknown peptide
4. Neuroendocrine-induced vasoconstriction
5. Endothelial cell relaxing factor
6. Microvascular infarction

Mechanism of Action of ACE Inhibitors. A review of formal studies of vasodilators does not provide strong evidence that these drugs are efficacious in the treatment of chronic heart failure [39]. This contrasts with the evidence showing considerable benefit from ACE inhibitors. It may be that the trials on ACE inhibitors were undertaken more recently, were better designed and included greater patient numbers. Many authors have assumed that the beneficial effect of ACE inhibition is due to vasodilatation resulting in improved function of the heart, regression of hypertrophy and possibly remodelling of the myocardium. An alternative mechanism is that ACE inhibitors are synergistic with diuretics to increase the loss of sodium and water. ACE inhibitors cause a diuresis if given acutely provided the perfusion pressure does not fall. The body sodium is then redistributed. The resistance to blood flow in the vasculature of exercising skeletal muscle would fall because of a reduction of intracellular sodium and relaxation of smooth muscle. Such an explanation easily accounts for the slow onset of clinical benefit after the initiation of therapy with ACE inhibitors.

Practical Implications for Treatment

An important distinction must be made between drugs often considered under the generic label "vasodilator drugs". All vasodilators are not the same. This author believes that ACE inhibitors should not even be classified as vasodilators.

The initial enthusiasm for vasodilator drugs has waned with the realisation that the immediate haemodynamic effects are often not sustained in the long term, do not relate to long-term clinical improvement of the patient, and the often dramatic acute haemodynamic changes do not bring about an increase of exercise capacity [25, 40].

Some vasodilators, possibly the nitrates, can be used with the intention of delaying the progression of damage to the myocadium although the mechanism is most uncertain. The evidence that vasodilators, nitrates and hydralazine alter mortality is weak [41].

The case for treating patients with heart failure with an ACE inhibitor is strong [15, 33, 34]. Symptoms are reduced, exercise capacity [33, 34, 42, 43] is increased, possibly the progression of damage is delayed [20], and mortality is altered favourably [15]. These findings apply to patients with severe heart failure almost regardless of aetiology. The major problem facing the clinician at the present time is how early in the natural history of heart failure to introduce ACE inhibitors, and whether patients with ventricular dysfunction should be treated. These issues may be resolved when the results of current trials are known.

Patients with mild heart failure [44] in contrast to those with severe heart failure [45] do not have elevation of the renin-angiotensin system until they are treated with diuretics. The logic for treating ventricular dysfunction is therefore not strong unless the effect is on the intracellular renin-angiotensin system and possibly on the processes concerned with reshaping and remodelling the heart. However, it would be rational to prescribe an ACE inhibitor whenever a diuretic is used to prevent the activation of the renin-angiotensin system. Trials in mild heart failure do show clinical benefit with the introduction of ACE inhibitors [42, 43]. Evidence shows that once patients have had an episode of sodium retention an ACE inhibitor is not adequate treatment [46]; a diuretic should be prescribed in addition.

Thus ACE inhibitors should be considered in all patients with moderate or severe heart failure. There is a case for using an ACE inhibitor as adjunctive therapy whenever a diuretic is used to treat heart failure. Whether ACE inhibitors should be used when left ventricular dysfunction is present in the absence of heart failure is as yet unknown. The benefit of vasodilators, such as nitrates, prazosin or hydralazine and excluding the ACE inhibitors, has not yet been shown to be of substantial clinical importance.

References

1. Cohn JN, Franciosa JA (1977) Vasodilator therapy of cardiac failure, pt. 1. N Engl J Med 297:27–31
2. Zelis R, Flaim SF, Moskowitz RM, Nellis SH (1979) How much can we expect from vasodilator therapy in congestive heart failure? Circulation 59:1092–1097
3. Braunwald E, Colucci WS (1984) Vasodilator therapy of heart failure. Has the promissory note been paid? N Engl J Med 310(7):459–461
4. Poole-Wilson PA (1985) Heart failure. Med Int 2:866–871
5. Poole-Wilson PA (1987) The management and treatment of chronic heart failure. In: Daswon AM, Besser GM (eds) Recent advances in medicine, vol. 20. Churchill Livingstone, Edinburgh, pp 161–175
6. Poole-Wilson PA (1984) The role of digitalis in the future. Br J Clin Pharmacol 18:1515–1565
7. Poole-Wilson PA (1988) Digitalis: dead or alive? Cardiology 75 [Suppl 1]:103–109
8. Anand IS, Veall N, Kalra GS, Ferrari R, Sutton G, Harris P, Poole-Wilson PA (1989) Treatment of heart failure with diuretics: body compartments, renal function and plasma hormones. Eur Heart J 10:445–450
9. Linzbach AJ (1960) Heart failure from the point of view of quantitative anatomy. Am J Cardiol 5:370–380
10. Soufer R, Wohlgelernter D, Vita NA, Amuchestegui M, Sostman D, Berger HJ, Zaret BL (1985) Intact systolic left ventricular function in clinical congestive heart failure. Am J Cardiol 55:1032–1036
11. Dougherty AH, Naccarelli GV, Gray EL, Hicks CH, Goldstein RA (1984) Congestive heart failure with normal systolic function. Am J Cardiol 54:778–782

12. Lavine SJ, Krishnaswami V, Shreiner DP, Amidi M (1985) Left ventricular diastolic filling in patients with left ventricular dysfunction. Int J Cardiol 8:423–436
13. Katz AM (1987) Role of the basic sciences in the practice of cardiology. J Mol Cell Cardiol 19:3–17
14. Henderson Y (1923) Volume changes of the heart. Physiol Rev 3:165–208
15. CONSENSUS Trial Study Group (1987) Effects of enalapril on mortality in severe congestive heart failure. Results of the Cooperative North Scandinavian Enalapril Survival Study (CONSENSUS). N Engl J Med 316:1429–1435
16. Franciosa JA, Willen M, Ziesche S, Cohn JN (1983) Survival in men with severe chronic left ventricular failure due to either coronary heart disease or idiopathic dilated cardiomyopathy. Am J Cardiol 51:831–836
17. Kannel WB, Plehn JF, Cupples LA (1988) Cardiac failure and sudden death in the Framingham Study. Am Heart J 115:869–875
18. Pfeffer J, Pfeffer MA, Braunwald E (1985) Influence of chronic captopril therapy on the infarcted left ventricle of the rat. Circ Res 57:84–95
19. Pfeffer MA, Lamas GA, Vaughan DE, Parisi AF, Braunwald E (1988) Effect of captopril on progressive ventricular dilatation after anterior myocardial infarction. N Engl J Med 319:80–86
20. Sharpe N, Murphy J, Smith H, Hannan S (1988) Treatment of patients with symptomless left ventricular dysfunction after myocardial infarction. Lancet i:255–259
21. Packer M (1985) Sudden unexpected death in patients with congestive heart failure: a second frontier. Circulation 72(4):681–685
22. Lipkin DP, Poole-Wilson PA (1986) Symptoms limiting exercise in chronic heart failure. Br Med J 292:1030–1031
23. Lipkin DP, Canepa-Anson R, Stephens MR, Poole-Wilson PA (1986) Factors determining symptoms in heart failure: comparison of fast and slow exercise tests. Br Heart J 55:439–445
24. Bayliss J, Canepa-Anson R, Norell MS, Poole-Wilson PA, Sutton G (1986) Vasodilatation with captopril and prazosin in chronic heart failure: double-blind study at rest and on exercise. Br Heart J 55:265–273
25. Franciosa JA, Goldsmith SR, Cohn JN (1980) Contrasting immediate and longterm effects of isosorbide dinitrate on exercise capacity in congestive heart failure. Am J Cardiol 69:559–566
26. Topic N, Kramer B, Massie B (1982) Acute and long-term effects of captopril on exercise cardiac performance and exercise capacity in congestive heart failure. Am Heart J 104:1172–1179
27. Siskind SJ, Sonnenblick EH, Forman R, Schever J, LeJemtel TH (1981) Acute substantial benefit of inotropic therapy with amrinone on exercise hemodynamics and metabolism in severe congestive heart failure. Circulation 64:966–973
28. Wade OL, Bishop JM (1962) Cardiac output and regional blood flow. Blackwell, Oxford
29. Zelis R, Flaim SF (1982) Alterations in vasomotor tone in congestive heart failure. Prog Cardiovasc Dis XXIV(6):437–459
30. LeJemtel TH, Maskin CS, Lucido D, Chadwick BJ (1986) Failure to augment limb blood flow in response to one-leg versus two-leg exercise in patients with severe heart failure. Circulation 74:245–251
31. Mancini DM, Davis L, Wexler JP, Chadwick B. LeJemtel TH (1987) Dependence of enhanced maximal exercise performance on increased peak skeletal muscle perfusion during long-term captopril therapy. J Am Coll Cardiol 10:845–850
32. Drexler H, Banhardt U, Meinertz T, Wollschlager H, Lehmann M, Just H (1989) Contrasting peripheral short-term and long-term effects of converting enzyme inhibition in patients with congestive heart failure. Circulation 79:491–502
33. Captopril Multicentre Research Group (1983) A placebo controlled trial of captopril in refractory chronic heart failure. J Am Coll Cardiol 2:755–763
34. Lipkin DP, Jones DA, Round JM, Poole-Wilson PA (1988) Abnormalities of skeletal muscle in patients with chronic heart failure. Int J Cardiol 18:187–195
35. Dunnigan A, Staley NA, Smith SA, Pierpont ME, Judd D, Benditt DG, Benson DW (1987) Cardiac and skeletal muscle abnormalities in cardiomyopathy: comparison of patients with ventricular tachycardia or congestive heart failure. J Am Coll Cardiol 10:608–618

36. Drexler H, Hiroi M, Riede U, Banhardt U, Meinertz T, Just H (1988) Skeletal muscle blood flow, metabolism and morphology in chronic congestive heart failure and effects of short and long term angiotensin-converting enzyme inhibition. Am J Cardiol 62:82E–85E
37. Wiener DH, Fink LI, Maris J, Jones RA, Chance B, Wilson JR (1986) Abnormal skeletal muscle bioenergetics during exercise in patients with heart failure: role of reduced muscle blood flow. Circulation 73:1127–1136
38. Massie BM, Conway M, Rajagopalan B, Yonge R, Frostick S, Ledingham J, Sleight P, Radda G (1988) Skeletal muscle metabolism during exercise under ischaemic conditions in congestive heart failure. Evidence for abnormalities unrelated to blood flow. Circulation 78:320–326
39. Lipkin DP, Poole-Wilson PA (1985) Treatment of chronic heart failure: a review of recent trials. Br Med J 291:993–996
40. Packer M, Lee WH, Kessler PD, Gottlieb SS, Medina N, Yushak M (1987) Prevention and reversal of nitrate tolerance in patients with congestive heart failure. N Engl J Med 317:799–804
41. Cohn JN, Archibald DG, Ziescah S, Franciosa JA, Harston WE, Tristani WE, Dunkman WB, Kacobs W, Francis GS, Flohr KH, Goldman S, Cobb FR, Shah PM, Saunders R, Fletcher RD, Loeb HS, Hughes VC, Baker B (1986) Effect of vasodilator therapy on mortality in chronic congestive heart failure. Results of a Veterans Administration Cooperative Study. N Engl J Med 314:1547–1552
42. Captopril-Digoxin Multicenter Research Group (1988) Comparative effects of therapy with captopril and digoxin in patients with mild to moderate heart failure. JAMA 259:539–544
43. German and Austrian Xamoterol Study Group (1988) Double-blind placebo-controlled comparison of digoxin and xamoterol in chronic heart failure. Lancet i:489–493
44. Bayliss J, Norell M, Canepa-Anson R, Sutton G, Poole-Wilson P (1987) Untreated heart failure: clinical and neuroendocrine effects of introducing diuretics. Br Heart J 57:17–22
45. Anand IS, Ferrari R, Kalra GS, Wahi PL, Poole-Wilson PA, Harris P (1989) Edema of cardiac origin: studies of body water and sodium, renal function, hemodynamics and plasma hormones in untreated congestive heart failure. Circulation 80:299–305
46. Richardson A, Bayliss J, Scriven AJ, Parameshwar J, Poole-Wilson PA, Sutton G (1987) Double-blind comparison of captopril alone against furosemide plus amiloride in mild heart failure. Lancet ii:709–711

Possible Role of Positive Inotropic Drugs in Congestive Heart Failure and in Left Ventricular Dysfunction

H. POULEUR

Introduction

Congestive heart failure is a complex clinical syndrome, in the pathophysiology of which several vicious circles and detrimental adaptive mechanisms (e.g., afterload mismatch, functional mitral regurgitation, activation of the renin-angiotensin, and sympathetic nervous systems) are involved. In recent years therapeutic successes have been achieved mainly with interventions interferring with the indirect consequences of heart failure such as vasoconstriction and renin activation. Besides symptomatic benefit, improved survival has been reported with the association of isosorbide dinitrate and hydralazine [1] and with the angiotensin converting enzyme inhibitor enalapril in New York Heart Association class IV heart failure patients [2].

The direct cause of heart failure, however, remains the systolic and/or diastolic dysfunction of the myocardium. In heart failure with important systolic dysfunction, the most logical therapeutic step would be to improve the contractile performance of the failing heart, i.e., to use a positive inotropic drug. The past decade has witnessed intense basic and clinical research in this field of positive inotropic drugs. So far, most results appear very disappointing. The purpose of this review is to examine the possible reasons underlying the lack of benefit of most positive inotropic drugs before discussing their possible role and directions for future research.

Difference Between a Positive Inotropic Agent and a Positive Inotropic Drug to Treat Chronic Heart Failure

An agent is said to have a positive inotropic action when it increases both the extent of shortening and the speed of myocardial shortening when all other factors affecting myocardial performance (preload, afterload, frequency of stimulation, synchrony, etc.) are kept constant [3]. Many compounds exhibit a positive inotropic effect when administered to normal mammalian myocardium, and some, like norepinephrine, have a major physiologic role.

A positive inotropic *drug* to treat chronic systolic myocardial failure, on the other hand, should be able to improve the contractility of the failing myocardium during prolonged administration. Research and development programs in the pharmaceutical industry failed to recognize this important distinction and screened their compounds on various animal models with a normal myocardium or, at best, on oversimplified models of acute heart failure such as ethanol or barbiturate intoxication.

The positive inotropic drug most likely to succeed is one that would specifically correct the abnormalities responsible for the systolic dysfunction. As we observe below, such a drug might have no positive inotropic effect at all on a normal myocardium, and it might even behave as a negative inotropic agent in the normal heart. In contrast to others [4], we do not believe that a useful positive inotrope must necessarily have clear-cut positive inotropic effects in the normal heart and in healthy volunteers. In our opinion, therefore, there is a need for seriously reconsidering the definition of a positive inotropic drug when discussing the future of this class of compounds.

Importance of the Clinical Setting and of the Therapeutic Goal

When trying to define the possible role of positive inotropic agents, it is useful to consider three different clinical settings. The first is the immediate life-saving situation as it may be encountered after cardiac surgery or in intensive care. In this setting, there is a definite role for powerful intravenous agents such as dopamine, dobutamine, and enoximone. This is particularly true when the cause of the depression in myocardial function is expected to be reversible and is related primarily to an abnormality in excitation-contraction coupling [5, 6]. A left ventricle with a large mass of "stunned myocardium" or some cases of acute intoxication may fall into this category.

The second setting is that of the chronic congestive heart failure, ranging in severity from functional class II to the patients who remain in class IV despite full therapy with diuretics, vasodilators, and angiotensin converting enzyme inhibitors. The aim of the therapy is at least to improve the symptoms and quality of life and, if possible, to improve survival. Cardiac glycosides, and more particularly digoxin, are used worldwide, but their clinical efficacy in patients in sinus rhyhtm has been repeatedly questioned. There is some evidence that in vitro ouabain is still able to produce a positive inotropic effect in human myocardium with end-stage failure [7], but this requires high, toxic concentrations. In some recent controlled trials, such as the captopril-digoxin trial [8], the milrinone-digoxin trial [9], and the German-Austrian xamoterol-digoxin trial [10], the trend was toward an improvement in exercise tolerance with digoxin. Other small controlled trials also suggested a functional benefit in patients in whom systolic dysfunction was the primary cause of the symptomatology. With respect to the effects of digoxin on cardiac mortality, on the other hand, the controversy continues, all studies being retrospective and uncontrolled [11]. The Clinical Trial Branch of the National Heart Lung and Blood Institute is planning a multicenter placebo-controlled study to evaluate the effects of digitalis on mortality in congestive heart failure. As long as the results of this study are not known, the presently available data suggest that digoxin remains a useful, although weak and with a low therapeutic index, positive inotrope [12] even in patients with sinus rhythm.

In the late 1970s, phosphodiesterase (PDE) III inhibitors such as amrinone and milrinone, rapidly followed by 10 to 15 other derivatives, were proposed as alternatives to cardiac glycosides. Despite a promising profile in the intact circulation (positive inotropic effect, improved relaxation, balanced veno- and arteriodilatation), the clinical results during prolonged therapy in mild to severe heart failure were appallingly negative: side-effects, arrhythmias, increased mortality, lack of functional benefit. For example, in 230 patients in sinus rhythm randomized to digoxin, milrinone, or the combination digoxin/milrinone, there was no significant benefit of milrinone over digoxin in terms of exercise tolerance. Ejection fraction was unchanged with milrinone but improved slightly with digoxin, and there were significantly more arrhythmias and side effects in the milrinone group. Further, the data suggested an increased mortality rate in the group treated with milrinone ($p<0.064$) [9]. We will not review further all published trials but rather examine the rationale for these poor results.

In mild to moderate heart failure, when intracellular cyclic AMP generation is still satisfactory, these agents increase intracellular cyclic-AMP which in a first step may improve contractility and relaxation but may also trigger arrhythmias, deplete the high-energy phosphate stores [13] and also accelerate the desensitization and down-regulation of the β-adrenoceptors [14]. Thus, if the patient survives the early arrhythmias, the drug will progressively loose its efficacy because less and less cyclic-AMP will be available. As noted above, another mechanism by which these agents may be detrimental is the depletion in high-energy phosphate stores. The failing heart is an "energy-starved organ" [15] because of abnormalities in mitochondrial function and because of inadequate cellular perfusion. Measurements made in our laboratory using a model of chronic volume-overload myocardial failure showed that, in contrast to the normal myocardium, ATP stores became depleted during inotropic stimulation with either dobutamine or sulmazol [13]. Now that NMR spectroscopy is available for human studies, this aspect of the energy balance of the failing heart during inotropic stimulation is certainly worth checking in patients.

In end-stage heart faillure, there is a defect in cyclic-AMP production, the β-adrenoceptors are down-regulated [7, 16], and the PDE III inhibitors as well as the β-stimulants loose their efficacy. In our opinion therefore, PDE III inhibitors and β-receptor full agonists have no role in the long-term treatment of chronic heart failure. It is also suggested that some positive inotropic agents might increase the sensitivity of the contractile proteins to calcium. This seems at least one of the mechanisms involved in the inotropic action of the drug DPI 201-106 [17]. The price to pay for such a positive inotropic action is a delayed myocardial relaxation. In all situations where the rate of calcium reuptake is impaired [15] this might result in a detrimental alteration in diastolic function.

Several β-adrenoceptor partial agonists have also been proposed to treat heart failure. The data obtained after prenalterol were considered negative [18], but an improvement in symptoms and quality of life has recently been reported in patients with mild to moderate heart failure using xamoterol [10], a β_1-adrenoceptor agonist with less intrinsic sympathomimetic activity (ISA) than prenalterol [19].

With the use of a β-adrenoceptor partial agonist, however, we reach a critical limit in the definition of a positive inotrope. Xamoterol, when administered under baseline conditions in normal subjects or in patients with only modest changes in resting sympathetic drive, definitely acts as a positive inotropic drug [20] even during long-term administration [21]. When sympathetic drive is increased, such as during exercise or in patients with severe congestive heart failure, xamoterol acts as a β-antagonist [22, 23]. As one of the most consistent effects of this agent is to improve left ventricular diastolic function [20, 21, 24], controversy still exists regarding the mechanisms by which this drug improves symptoms and exercise tolerance in moderate heart failure.

Moreover, because of its antagonistic action, the administration of xamoterol may be potentially detrimental in class IV unstable heart failure. Interestingly, however, full $β_1$-adrenoceptor antagonists such as metoprolol have been used in dilated cardiomyopathy. Careful progressive dosing appears necessary, and only a subset of patients actually tolerates this therapy. As shown in Table 1, several studies have been performed using this approach [25–32], and in some of these an improvement in left ventricular function was observed during long-term treatment. Recently, it was shown that this improvement was accompanied by an increased density in $β_1$-adrenoceptors and by a restoration of the responsiveness to sympathetic stimulation [32]. Obviously, the total experience with this therapeutic approach is limited, and patients with dilated cardiomyopathy might represent a different entity from the most common form of heart failure, ischemic heart disease, where myocardial destruction is generally extensive and irreversible. Nevertheless, the changes in myocardial performance observed in some patients after long-term metoprolol therapy are consistent with a positive inotropic effect [32]. Thus, we have an example of a drug that may act in a subset of heart failure patients as a real positive inotropic drug even though its acute effects and its effects on the normal heart are quite different. This should encourage research at least to explore new avenues and to try to define better the biochemical mechanisms responsible for the depressed contractility rather than naively screening for compounds that increase dP/dt_{max} in normal anesthetized animals.

A third potential indication for positive inotropes would be the patients with asymptomatic left ventricular dysfunction. The hope in this case would be to prevent or at least to delay the relentless progression of the left ventricular dysfunction toward congestive heart failure. A similar approach is now being attempted using angiotensin-converting enzyme inhibitors. It has been proposed that increased diastolic wall stress was one of the factors involved in the remodeling of the left ventricle after acute myocardial infarction, and that in some cases remodeling was inadequate and led to late heart failure. Xamoterol produces substantial reduction in diastolic wall stress, and preliminary data suggest that this agent might indeed influence the remodeling of the left ventricle during prolonged therapy [24]. Further studies are obviously needed to confirm these results, to determine the optimal timing of the therapy, and, more importantly, to establish the long-term benefit for the patient.

In conclusion, the alterations in systolic performance in congestive heart failure have various etiologies, some of which cannot be improved by positive

Table 1. Summary of results of studies using β-blockers in patients with congestive heart failure (CHF)

Reference	Study design	n	Cause of CHF	β-Blocker	Mean follow-up	Effects on CHF
Waagstein et al. [25]	Open, uncontrolled	7	IDCM	Practolol (6) Alprenolol (1)	5 months	Overall improvement in symptoms, exercise, LV function
Swedberg et al. [26]	Open, uncontrolled	28	IDCM	Metoprolol (17) Alprenolol (7) Practolol (2) Propranolol (2)	23 months	Improved EF from 0.32 ± 0.02 to 0.42 ± 0.04, improved NYHA class, lower mortality
Ikram and Fitzpatrick [27]	Double-blind crossover	15	IDCM (4) alcoholic (11)	Acebutolol or placebo	1 month	No change in EF or NYHA class, CT ratio and exercise time worsened
Currie et al. [28]	Double-blind crossover	10	IDCM (4 also CAD)	Metoprolol or placebo	1 month	No change in EF, NYHA class, exercise tolerance, CI worsened
Engelmeier et al. [29]	Double-blind randomized	37	IDCM	Metoprolol or placebo	12 months 10 months	Improved EF (16), NYHA class (8), exercise tolerance (8)
Anderson et al. [30]	Double-blind randomized	50	IDCM	Metoprolol or placebo	19 months	Improved NYHA class, exercise, survival
Gilbert et al. [31]	Randomized	15	IDCM	Bucindolol (9) or placebo	2 months	Significant improvements in EF, HR, LVSWI, PW, CI
Heilbrunn et al. [32]	Open, uncontrolled	14	IDCM	Metoprolol	6 months	Improved hemodynamics, EF, response to dobutamine, β-receptor density

IDCM, Idiopathic dilated cardiomyopathy; EF, ejection fraction; CT, cardiothoracic.

inotropic drugs, such as the destruction by a myocardial infarction or the impaired perfusion. The biochemical abnormalities responsible for the depressed contractility, on the other hand, are complex and are still poorly understood. They probably involve alterations in the receptor population and regulatory proteins [14, 16], in the properties of the sarcolemma and the sarcoplasmic reticulum, and in mitochondrial function [15]. Alterations in structural proteins and enzyme synthesis may also be present. It is obviously desirable to correct these abnormalities once identified, and the drug able to accomplish this feat will probably improve myocardial performance, i.e., it will behave as a positive inotropic drug. There is therefore a definite role for positive inotropic agents in the treatment of heart failure. The compounds likely to succeed, however, are not yet available, and as long as research on inotropes is not more sharply focused on the chronically failing heart rather than on the normal heart, pharmaceutical companies are likely to fail.

Acknowledgement. The author thanks Mrs. Isabelle Mottard for her excellent secretarial assistance.

References

1. Cohn JN, Archibald DG, Ziesche S, Franciosa JA, Harston WE, Tristani FE, Dunkman WB, Jacobs W, Francis GS, Flohr KH, Goldman S, Cobb FR, Shah PM, Saunders R, Flecher RD, Loeb HS, Hughes VC, Baker B (1986) Effect of vasodilator therapy on mortality in chronic congestive heart failure. Results of a Veteran Administration Cooperative Study. N Engl J Med 314:1547–1552
2. CONSENSUS Trial Study Group (1987) Effects of enalapril on mortality in severe congestive heart failure. Results of the Cooperative North Scandinavian Enalapril Survival Study (CONSENSUS). N Engl J Med 316:1429–1435
3. Braunwald E, Ross J Jr, Sonnenblick EH (1976) Methods for assessing cardiac contractility. In: Mechanisms of contraction of the normal and failing heart. Braunwald E et al. (eds) Little Brown, Boston, pp 130–165
4. Braunwald E, Colucci WS (1984) Evaluating the efficacy of new inotropic agents. J Am Coll Cardiol 3:1570–1574
5. Braunwald E, Kloner RA (1982) The stunned myocardium: prolonged, postischemic ventricular dysfunction. Circulation 66:1146–1149
6. Schaper W, Ito B, Buchwald A, Tate H, Schaper J (1986) Molecular and ultrastructural basis of left ventricular reperfusion dysfunction. Adv Cardiol 34:1–15
7. Feldman MD, Copelas L, Gwathmey JK, Phillips P, Warren SE, Schoen FJ (1987) Deficient production of cyclic AMP: pharmacologic evidence of an important cause of contractile dysfunction in patients with end-stage heart failure. Circulation 75:331–339
8. Captopril-Digoxin group (1988) Comparative effects of therapy with captopril and digoxin in patients with mild to moderate heart failure. JAMA 259:539–544
9. De Bianco R, Shabetai R, Kostuk W, Moran J, Schlant R, Wright R for the Milrinone Multicenter group (1989) A comparison of oral milrinone, digoxin and their combination in the treatment of patients with chronic heart failure. N Engl J Med 320:677–683
10. German and Austrian Xamoterol Study Group (1988) Double-blind placebo controlled comparison of digoxin and xamoterol in chronic heart failure. Lancet i:489–493
11. Yusuf S, Wittes J, Bailey K, Furberg C (1986) Digitalis – a new controversy regarding an old drug. The pitfalls of inappropriate methods. Circulation 73:14–18
12. Cohn J (1989) Inotropic therapy for heart failure. Paradise postponed. N Engl J Med 320:729–731

13. Pouleur H, Marechal G, Balasim H, Van Mechelen H, Ries A, Rousseau MF, Charlier AA (1983) Effects of dobutamine and sulmazol (AR-L115 BS) on myocardial metabolism, coronary, femoral and renal blood flows: a comparative study in normal dogs and in dogs with chronic volume overload. J Cardiovasc Pharmacol 5:861–867
14. Strasser RH, Krimmer J, Marquetant R (1988) Regulation of β-adrenergic receptors: impaired desensitization in myocardial ischemia. J Cardiovasc Pharmacol 12:S15–S24
15. Katz AM (1988) Cellular mechanisms in congestive heart failure. Am J Cardiol 62:3A–8A
16. Bristow MR, Ginsburg R, Umans V, Fowler M, Minobe W, Rasmussen R, Zera P, Menlove R, Shah P, Jamieson S, Stinson EB (1986) β_1- and β_2-adrenergic-receptor subpopulations in nonfailing and failing human ventricular myocardium: coupling of both receptor subtypes to muscle contraction and selective β_1-receptor down-regulation in heart failure. Circ Res 59:297–309
17. Hajjar RJ, Gwathmey JK, Briggs GM, Morgan JP (1988) Differential effect of DPI 201-206 on control and myopathic heart muscle. J Clin Invest 82:1578–1584
18. Lambertz H, Meyer J, Erbel R (1984) Long-term hemodynamic effects of prenalterol in patients with severe congestive heart failure. Circulation 69:298–305
19. Nuttall A, Snow HM (1982) The cardiovascular effects of ICI 118,587: a β_1-adrenoceptor partial agonist. Br J Pharmacol 77:381–388
20. Rousseau MF, Pouleur H, Vincent MF (1983) Effects of a cardioselective beta$_1$-partial agonist (Corwin) on left ventricular function and myocardial metabolism in patients with previous myocardial infarction. Am J Cardiol 51:1267–1274
21. Pouleur H, Etienne J, Van Mechelen H, Gurné O, Rousseau MF (1990) Effects of the β_1-adrenoceptor partial agonist xamoterol on the left ventricular diastolic function: an evaluation after 1 to 6 years of oral therapy. Circulation 81(III): 87–92
22. Sato H, Inoue M, Matsuyama T, Ozaki H, Shimazu T, Takeda H, Ishida Y, Kamada T (1987) Hemodynamic effects of the β_1-adrenoceptor partial agonist xamoterol in relation to plasma norepinephrine levels during exercise in patients with left ventricular dysfunction. Circulation 75:213–220
23. Detry JM, Decoster PM, Brasseur LA (1983) Hemodynamic effects of Corwin (ICI 118,587), a new cardioselective beta-adrenoceptor partial agonist. Eur Heart J 4:584–591
24. Pouleur H, van Eyll C, Hanet C, Cheron P, Charlier AA, Rousseau MF (1988) Long-term effects of xamoterol on left ventricular diastolic function and late remodeling: a study in patients with anterior myocardial infarction and single-vessel disease. Circulation 77:1081–1089
25. Waagstein F, Hjalmarson A, Varnauskas E, Wallentin I (1975) Effect of chronic β-adrenergic receptor blockade in congestive cardiomyopathy. Br Heart J 37:1022–1036
26. Swedberg K, Hjalmarson A, Waagstein F, Wallentin I (1980) Beneficial effects of long-term β-blockade in congestive cardiomyopathy. Br Heart J 44:117–133
27. Ikram H, Fitzpatrick D (1981) Double-blind trial of chronic oral β-blockade in congestive cardiomyopathy. Lancet ii:490–493
28. Currie PJ, Kelly MJ, McKenzie A (1984) Oral β-adrenergic blockade with metoprolol in chronic severe dilated cardiomyopathy. J Am Coll Cardiol 3:203–209
29. Engelmeier RS, O'Connell JB, Walsh R, Rad N, Scanlon PJ, Gunnar RM (1985) Improvement in symptoms and exercise tolerance by metoprolol in patients with dilated cardiomyopathy: a double-blind, randomized, placebo-controlled trial. Circulation 72:536–546
30. Anderson JL, Lutz JR, Gilbert EM, Sorensen SG, Yanowitz FG, Menlove RL, Bartholomew M (1985) A randomized trial of low-dose β-blockade therapy for idiopathic dilated cardiomyopathy. Am J Cardiol 55:471–475
31. Gilbert EM, Anderson JL, Deitchman D (1987) Chronic β-blockade with bucindolol improves resting cardiac function in dilated cardiomyopathy. Circulation 76:IV-358
32. Heilbrunn SM, Shah P, Bristow MR, Valantine HA, Ginsburg R, Fowler MB (1989) Increased β-receptor density and improved hemodynamic response to catecholamine stimulation during long-term metoprolol therapy in heart failure from dilated cardiomyopathy. Circulation 79:483–490

Prognostic Indices and Prolongation of Life

K. Swedberg

Introduction

Patients with congestive heart failure have an unfavorable prognosis. The Framingham Study reported the natural history in patients developing heart failure between 1949 and 1965 [1]. The survival rates after 1 and 5 years were 79% and 38% in men and 86% and 57% in women, respectively. Whether the natural history has changed since then is unclear, and the prognosis remains ominous. There are number of reports from referral institutions in recent years also demonstrating a high mortality, with 1-year survival in the range of 50% [2]. In the clinical situation as well as in the evaluation of therapeutic interventions there is an interest in estimating the patient's prognosis. It is the aim of this paper to review some prognostic indices and to discuss whether survival in congestive heart failure has improved with respect to these indices.

From the literature regarding prognostic information in heart failure, data have emerged that may justify classification of the prognostic indicators into four groups: clinical symptomatology, myocardial function, ventricular arrhythmias, and neuroendocrine activation.

Clinical Symptomatology

It is a well-recognized clinical experience that markedly symptomatic patients have a worse long-term survival than less symptomatic patients; this has been documented in several studies [3–5]. However, as can be seen in Fig. 1, patients in NYHA classes II and III have a similar 1 year mortality of around 20%; patients in NYHA class IV have a significantly lower survival with 1 year mortality of around 50%–60% [4]. Stability of symptoms also seems to be of importance. Patients showing progressive clinical deterioration have a significantly lower survival rate than those with more stable symptoms [3].

One study has evaluated prognostic effects of therapy in relation to NYHA class. In the CONSENSUS study all patients were in NYHA class IV at randomization [6]. The only objective requirement in this study was a dilated heart on chest X-ray. The 127 patients randomized to receive placebo therapy in addition to optimal treatment including diuretics and vasodilators had a 6-month mortality of 49% based on life-table estimation. In patients randomized to enalapril

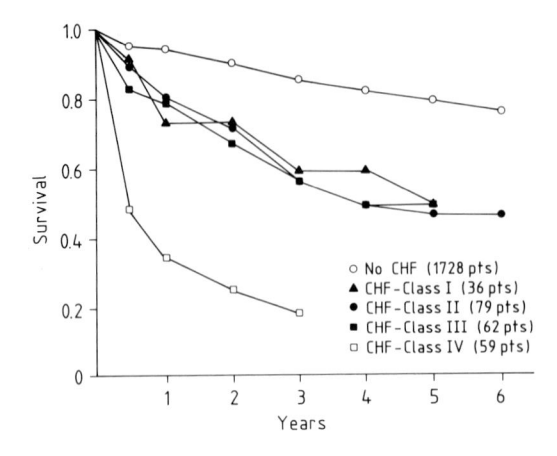

Fig. 1. Survival in relation to clinical symptoms according to New York Heart Association. *CHF*, Congestive heart failure. (Reproduced with permission from Califf et al. [4])

therapy the mortality was reduced significantly by 40% from 48% to 29%. Even if the enalapril-treated patients survived much longer, they still demonstrate a high mortality rate.

Myocardial Function

There have been many attempts to describe myocardial function. The most commonly used in the clinical situation is ejection fraction. This has also been used as a selection criteria in many studies. The value of a reduced ejection fraction as a prognostic marker has been clearly demonstrated [7]. However, as ejection fraction in most cases expresses volume changes according to Starling's law, it should be more accurate to measure left ventricular volumes. This has also been demonstrated by White et al. [8]. In a follow-up of consecutive patients undergoing coronary angiography after myocardial infarction, it was shown that end-systolic volume followed by end-diastolic volume were the most significant predictors of long-term prognosis out of a number of indicators of myocardial function (Fig. 2). Ejection fraction was also a predictor, but the volume measurements could be used within different ranges of ejection fraction.

In a number of studies different hemodynamic variables, such as cardiac index, stroke work index, and left ventricular filling pressure, have been used as predictors of outcome. Unfortunately, there is a large variation leading to an uncertainty in the clinical situation.

Recently, an interesting prognostic indicator has been described by Tan [9]. The maximal power output from the heart could clearly separate between survivors and nonsurvivors. The power output in Watts was calculated from cardiac output and developed arterial pressure during exercise. Tan also demonstrated that exercise could be replaced by a maximal inotropic stimulation by dobutamine [10]. This interesting observation remains to be validated.

As a reduced myocardial function predicts a poor long-term survival, it seems natural to try to improve the pumping function and hope that this translates into

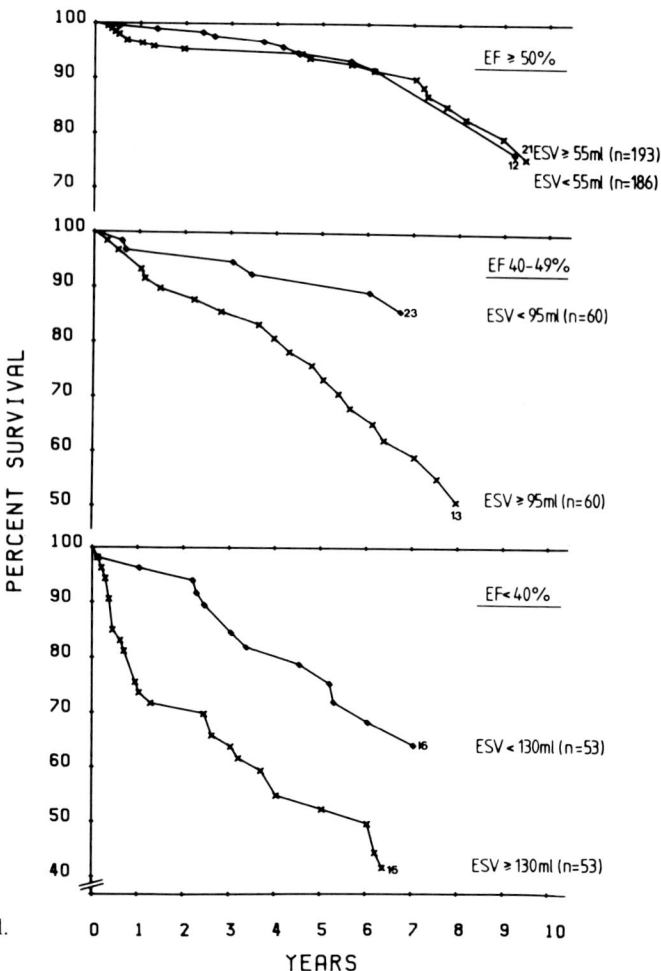

Fig. 2. Survival in relation to end-systolic volumes (*ESV*). *EF*, Ejection fraction. (Reproduced with permission from White et al. [8])

increased survival. However, in spite of many efforts the use of inotropic agents has not been shown to prolong survival in patients with congestive heart failure. On the contrary, there are indications that this mode of therapy even increases mortality [11–13]. Presently, there are ongoing studies that hopefully will clarify this important question.

Ventricular Arrhythmias

Complex ventricular arrhythmias have been demonstrated to be associated with increased mortality in several studies [14]. This is also true in congestive heart failure where serious arrhythmias are related to sudden death [5] as well reduced survival. In heart failure the question of arrhythmias as prognostic indicators is more complex because of the association between myocardial function, therapy, and serious ventricular arrhythmias. Bigger et al. have shown that an ejection fraction below 30% is associated with significantly more complex ventricular arrhythmias than a higher ejection fraction [15]. This finding has also been reported by Dargie et al. [16]. Furthermore, they demonstrated a relationship between arrhythmias and abnormalities in serum electrolytes. Hypokalemia and hyponatremia could be induced by intense pharmacologic therapy and thus indirect markers of the heart failure.

The suppression of ventricular arrhythmias has obviously been most appealing in the efforts to prolong life in patients with congestive heart failure. In one open nonrandomized study amiodarone treatment was associated with improved survival [16]. However, other studies have not been able to demonstrate any improvement in survival from class I antiarrhythmic agents. On the contrary, the recently published CAST-trial could even show a significant excess mortality in patients who responded to encainide or flecainide, two effective antiarrhythmic agents belonging to class Ic [17]. Whether the results from CAST can be translated to patients with symptomatic serious ventricular arrhythmias is uncertain. From this trial it is clear that antiarrhythmic therapy should be administered to patients with congestive heart failure only when the arrhythmias are obviously life threatening.

Neuroendocrine Activation

During the development of congestive heart failure, compensatory systems are activated in order to maintain perfusion pressure and circulatory distribution. This activation of circulatory reflexes includes the activation of neuroendocrine mechanisms and the release of hormones that affect circulation: noradrenaline, adrenaline, angiotensin II, and aldosterone. In addition, another hormone involved in this hormonal activation with the objective of balancing the effects of the activation of the renin-angiotensin-aldosterone system is released from the atrial myocardium: atrial natriuretic peptide (ANP).

This hormonal activation has been considered beneficial and essential for patients with congestive heart failure. However, recent information seems to contradict this view. Activation of the sympathetic nervous system may be expressed by the plasma levels of noradrenaline. Cohn et al. have reported that plasma noradrenaline levels were the best prognostic indicator out of a number of hemodynamic measurements evaluated in 106 patients with advanced congestive heart failure [18].

The prognostic importance of electrolyte abnormalities has been studied by Lee and Packer [19]. They found that serum sodium was the most powerful prognostic predictor out of 30 variables in 203 patients with heart failure. Plasma noradrenaline was not evaluated in this report. Patients with normal serum sodium concentrations did significantly better than patients with hyponatremia. Serum sodium was significantly related to plasma renin activity ($r=0.68$).

Recently, the relationship between ANP and survival was described by Gottlieb et al. [20]. In 102 patients they found that a plasma ANP level above the median level of 125 pg/ml to be associated with significantly higher mortality than a lower level.

Hormonal assessments were also performed in the CONSENSUS trial in 239 out of the 253 randomized patients. As has been described above, these patients were all in NYHA functional class IV and treated with diuretics, and in 50% also with spironolactone. Among patients randomized to additional placebo treatment, there was a significant positive relationship between 6-month mortality and plasma levels of noradrenaline, adrenaline, angiotension II, aldosterone, or ANP [21]. The combined activation of these hormones was found to be even more predictive of mortality [22]. More extensive information on these studies is presently awaiting publication.

Accordingly, the compensatory activation of cardiovascular hormones may be deleterious for the patient in congestive heart failure [21]. The counteraction of this activation would then be beneficial. In a retrospective analysis we found that patients with idiopathic dilated cardiomyopathy had a significantly improved survival compared to controls if they were treated with beta blockade [23]. This controversial observation is presently under evaluation in the Metoprol in Dilated Cardiomyopathy trial, an international multicenter trial.

In their patients with hyponatremia Lee and Packer found that the prognosis was significantly improved if treatment with a converting enzyme inhibitor had been started [19]. From the CONSENSUS trial we have been able to demonstrate that the addition of enalapril significantly offset the relationship between hormonal levels and mortality. From these studies it seems that if patients with advanced heart failure are treated with an converting enzyme inhibitor, mortality is significantly reduced.

Summary

In congestive heart failure it is possible to estimate prognosis from clinical symptomatology, left ventricular volumes and ejection fraction, complex ventricular arrhythmias, and neuroendocrine activation. Prognostic improvement based on these predictors can be obtained by the addition of an angiotensin converting enzyme inhibitor. Inotropic agents and class I antiarrhythmic agents do not improve mortality and may even have deleterious long-term effects.

References

1. McKee PA, Castelli WP, McNamara PM, Kannel WB (1971) The natural history of congestive heart failure: the Framingham Study. N Engl J Med 285:1441
2. Massie BM, Conway M (1987) Survival of patients with congestive heart failure: past, present, and future prospects. Circulation 75 [Suppl IV]:IV-II
3. Massie B, Ports T, Chatterjee K et al. (1981) Long-term vasodilator therapy for heart failure: clinical response and its relationship to hemodynamic measurements. Circulation 63(2):269–278

4. Califf RM, Bounous P, Harrell FE et al. (1982) The prognosis in the presence of coronary artery disease. In: Braunwald E, Mock MB, Watson JT (ed) Congestive heart failure. Grune and Stratton, New York, pp 31–40
5. Wilson J, Schwartz JS, St John Sutton M et al. (1983) Prognosis in severe heart failure: relation to hemodynamic measurements and ventricular ectopic activity. J Am Coll Cardiol 2:403–410
6. The CONSENSUS Trial Study Group (1987) Effects of enalapril on mortality in severe congestive heart failure. Results of the Cooperative North Scandinavian Enalapril Survival Study (CONSENSUS). N Engl J Med 316:1429–1435
7. Hammermeister KE, DeRouen TA, Dodge T (1979) Selection by univariate and multivariate analyses from the clinical, electrocardiographic, exercise, arteriographic and quantitative angiographic evaluations. Circulation 59(3):421–430
8. White HD, Norris RM, Brown M et al. (1987) Left ventricular end-systolic volume as the major determinant of survival after recovery from myocardial infarction. Circulation 76(1):44–51
9. Tan LB (1986) Cardiac pumping capability and prognosis in heart failure. Lancet ii:1360–1363
10. Tan LB, Brain RJI, Littler WA (1989) Assessing cardiac pumping capability by exercise testing an inotropic stimulation. Br Heart J 62:20–25
11. Massie B (1988) Is neurohormonal activation deleterious to long-term outcome of patients with congestive heart failure? J Am Coll Cardiol 12(2):559–569
12. Cohn J (1989) Inotropic therapy for heart failure. Paradise postponed. Editorial. N Engl J Med 320(11):729–731
13. DiBianco R, Shabetai R, Kostuk W et al. (1989) A comparison of oral milrinone, digoxin and their combination in the treatment of patients with chronic heart failure. N Engl J Med 320(11):677–683
14. Follansbee WP, Michelsen EL, Morganroth J (1980) Nonsustained ventricular tachycardia in ambulatory patients: characteristics and association with sudden cardiac death. Ann Intern Med 92:741–747
15. Bigger JT, Fleiss JL, Kleiger R, Miller JP, Rolnitsky LM (1984) The relationships among ventricular arrhythmias, left ventricular dysfunction and mortality in the two years after myocardial infarction. Circulation 69:250–258
16. Dargie HJ, Cleland JGF, Leckie BJ (1987) Relation of arrhythmias and electrolyte abnormalities to survival in patients with severe chronic heart failure. Circulation 75 [Suppl IV]:IV-98
17. The Cardiac Arrhythmia Suppression Trial (CAST) Investigators (1989) Preliminary report: effect of encainide and flecainide on mortality in a randomized trial of arrhythmia suppression after myocardial infarction. N Engl J Med 321:406–412
18. Cohn JN, Levine TB, Olivari MT et al. (1984) Plasma norepinphrine as a guide to prognosis in patients with chronic congestive heart failure. N Engl J Med 311:819–823
19. Hung Lee W, Packer M (1986) Prognostic importance of serum sodium concentration and its modification by converting-enzyme inhibition in patients with severe chronic heart failure. Circulation 73(2):257–267
20. Gottlieb S, Kukin ML, Ahern D, Paker M (1989) Prognostic importance of atrial natriuretic peptide in patients with chronic heart failure. J Am Coll Cardiol 13:1534–1539
21. Swedberg K, Eneroth P, Kjekshus J, Wilhelmsen for the CONSENSUS Trial Study Group (1988) Plasma concentrations of hormones affecting cardiovascular function in relation to mortality in severe congestive heart failure. Circulation Suppl II-575
22. Swedberg K, Hjalmarsson A, Waagstein F, Wallentin I (1979) Prolongation of survival in congestive cardiomyopathy by beta-receptor blockade. Lancet ii:1374–1376
23. Swedberg K, Eneroth P, Kjekshus J et al. (1989) Cardiovascular hormones in relation to mortality in severe heart failure. J Am Coll Cardiol 13:246 A (abstract)

Antiarrhythmic Approach

Editorial:
Heart Failure and Malignant Ventricular Arrhythmias

A. J. CAMM

Arrhythmic death is thought to be common in patients with heart failure because about half of those who succumb die suddenly and because ventricular arrhythmias are commonplace in patients with heart failure. Although this has never been convincingly proven it is likely to be true, because fortuitous ECG monitoring at the moment of death usually demonstrates a ventricular arrhythmia. It remains possible, however, that such arrhythmias are an epiphenomenon rather than a direct cause of death. Final proof of the causal role of ventricular arrhythmias in the death of heart failure patients requires definitive results of specific antiarrhythmic treatment in a large group of suitable patients. As yet no such evidence exists, but the results of many relevant trials involving antiarrhythmic drugs or implantable cardioverter/defibrillators are expected soon.

Heart failure is associated with a high incidence of cardiac arrhythmias because the consequences – neuro-endocrine (e.g. activation of the sympathetic nervous system), metabolic (hypokalaemia) and mechanical (such as stretch) – of heart failure and its treatment are arrhythmogenic. Furthermore, the pathology responsible for the loss of myocardial contractile function, for example ischaemic or myopathic disease, may also create an arrhythmic substrate, and agents used to treat heart failure, such as digoxin and positive inotropic drugs, may have direct arrhythmic electrophysiological properties. The arrhythmia, especially when chronic, or at least incessant, may aggravate or cause heart failure. Atrial fibrillation, incessant supraventricular tachycardia and frequently repetitive ventricular tachyarrhythmias have all been incriminated.

It is far from clear which arrhythmias merit treatment in the context of heart failure (see Gorgels et al.). Obviously, those arrhythmias which provoke failure should be controlled. Ventricular arrhythmias which produce serious symptoms, such as syncope, demand urgent treatment in their own right. It is more difficult to decide upon treatment when the arrhythmias are asymptomatic or only mildly symptomatic. In such instances the reason for eradicating the arrhythmia lies in an attempt to reduce the risk of sudden death on the basis that the observed arrhythmia is a cause, or minor version, of a potentially fatal rhythm disturbance. However, there is no evidence to date that such a treatment is warranted.

To date, the essential electrophysiological and arrhythmic consequences of various forms of heart failure have not been well characterized and differentiated from the effects of the underlying pathology. Any improvement seen after the successful treatment of heart failure has not been separately atttributed to the improved haemodynamics rather than the direct effects of drugs used to achieve resolution of the heart failure. Although the effects of antiarrhythmic drugs on cardiac contractility and haemodynamics are well understood, the electrophysiological effects of anti-failure treatments are relatively unknown. Similarly, little is known about modification of antiarrhythmic or electrophysiologic effects of antiarrhythmic drugs in the presence of heart failure or heart failure treatments (see Brachmann et al.).

Despite the popular conviction that heart failure patients die arrhythmic deaths, no good data support the use of antiarrhythmic drug therapy in such patients. Encainide and flecainide were given to post-MI patients in the CAST study (see Woosley). The active treatment group fared badly by comparison with the placebo-treated patients. A proarrhythmic mechanism is proposed as the most likely cause of the relatively high mortality in the treated group. Proarrhythmia and aggravation of ventricular function is known to occur most commonly in those patients with left ventricular dysfunction, especially when serious ventricular arrhythmias are treated with class 1 drugs. Even in patients with atrial arrhythmias some seemingly harmless antiarrhythmic drugs have been associated with definite excess mortality. The possible advantageous effects of class 3 drugs such as amiodarone and sotalol have not been thoroughly explored in patients with left ventricular failure. Preliminary results with amiodarone in post-MI patients with depressed left ventricular function auger well, and large-scale definitive trials (Canadian-American Myocardial Infarction Amiodarone Trial [CAMIAT]), European Myocardial Infarction Amiodarone Trial [EMIAT] are now under way. In the one small study in patients with overt heart failure no improvement in mortality was associated with amiodarone treatment but, nevertheless, a definitive study is presently being undertaken by the Veterans Administration in the United States.

In view of the risk of proarrhythmia and aggravation of heart failure associated with antiarrhythmic drug treatment, it has been suggested that it might be better to explore the use of implantable defibrillators in patients with severe heart failure who have not yet presented with a serious arrhythmia (see Saksena). In patients with lethal arrhythmias, many of whom have severe left ventricular dysfunction and overt heart failure, the implantable defibrillator has already been shown to reduce loss of life considerably. Whatever treatment is considered as a means of reducing the high mortality associated with heart failure it must obviously be substantiated by means of a formal clinical trial of clear design and sufficient power. Such trials are under way with the implantable defibrillator, and results are expected in the early 1990's.

Heart Failure and Ventricular Arrhythmias – The Antiarrhythmic Approach

B. LÜDERITZ

The question of when to treat arrhythmia in heart failure was discussed by P. M. Gorgels, Maastricht, also on behalf of P. Brugada and H. J. J. Wellens (this volume). The authors feel that treatment of cardiac dysrhythmias in heart failure is indicated when the arrhythmia causes heart failure, presents sufficiently severe symptoms, or impairs prognosis. Based on the Cardiac Arrhythmia Suppression Trial (CAST), it should be emphasized that the benefit of antiarrhythmic drugs should be weighed against proarrhythmic effects, risk of extracardiac side effects, and the increased risk of heart failure.

R. L. Woosley, Washington D.C., presented the CAST study in detail (this volume). For patients with a history of congestive heart failure (CHF) and asymptomatic ventricular arrhythmias it was concluded that effective therapy of a patient's CHF will improve the quality of life and that therapy with angiotensin-converting enzyme inhibitors will decrease mortality.

The data from CAST and the limited data from other trials with patients suffering from CHF do not support the use of the local anesthetic class of antiarrhythmic drugs in these patients and actually suggest that some may be contraindicated. Until a clinical trial has been performed with such patients, the use of antiarrhythmic drugs must be considered an unproven benefit.

Symptomatic CHF was not an enrollment criterion for CAST, but all patients had some evidence of ventricular dysfunction: 50% of the patients had an ejection fraction less than 40%, and 15% had an ejection fraction less than 30%. The increased mortality was common to all groups in CAST, including those with decreased ventricular function, and is likely to be seen in patients with a history of congestive heart failure and asymptomatic ventricular arrhythmias (Woosley, this volume).

Based on CAST the question arises: Did the antiarrhythmic approach change after CAST? CAST was a multicenter, randomized, placebo controlled study designed to test whether the suppression of asymptomatic or mildly symptomatic ventricular arrhythmias after myocardial infarction would reduce the rate of death from arrhythmia [10]. An attempt was made to find the safest and most effective agents.

Since the Cardiac Arrhythmia Pilot Study (CAPS) had demonstrated high suppression rates and few side effects for encainide and flecainide (both class 1 c drugs) and moricizine (an investigational class 1 a agent) [9], patients were randomly assigned to placebo or to one of these antiarrhythmic drugs. Patients with an ejection fraction of less than 30% were not given flecainide because of its known negative inotropic effects. The safety of the trial was further enhanced by giving patients a drug only after demonstrating a reduction of at least 80% of the premature ventricular beats and of 90% of the episodes of ventricular tachycardia with that drug [3, 10]. The eligibility criterion of patients on the basis of the screening Holter recording was six or more ventricular premature depolarizations per hour. Because the risk of death from arrhythmia after a myocardial infarction decreases with time, and in order to enroll enough potentially high-risk patients to maintain adequate statistical power, a lower ejection fraction was required for patients whose myocardial infarction had occurred more than 90 days before Holter recording. If the qualifying Holter recording was obtained within 90 days of the myocardial infarction, a left ventricular ejection fraction of 55% or less was required. If the qualifying Holter recording was performed between 90 days and two years after the myocardial infarction, an ejection fraction of 40% or less was required. Patients were excluded if they had ventricular arrhythmias causing more severe symptoms (such as syncope or presyncope) resulting from hemodynamic compromise or if they had any unsustained ventricular tachycardia with 15 or more successive beats at a rate of >120 beats per minute. The study's Data and Safety Monitoring Board terminated the flecainide and encainide arms of the trial following the report of an increase in mortality in patients taking these drugs compared with that in controls.

On April 17, 1989, after examining preliminary data the safety committee for CAST found that 56 of 730 patients (7.7%) receiving encainide or flecainide for an average of 10 months had died, whereas among 725 patients on placebo only 22 (3%) had died; this represents a more than two-fold increase of mortality in the drug-treated patients. Investigators were advised on April 20, 1989, to stop administering the two drugs. The data for moricizine are not yet available, as the monitoring board has observed no statistically significant effect at this early point and the trial is continuing.

Based on the data of CAST, the Food and Drug Administration (FDA) has decided that the use of flecainide should be reserved for the management of life-threatening arrhythmias such as ventricular tachycardia.

The drug should not be used in patients with less severe arrhythmias even if they are symptomatic.

Although its basis is not entirely clear, the unexpected outcome of patients treated with flecainide or encainide is best explained as the result of the induction of lethal ventricular arrhythmias (i.e., a proarrhythmic effect of the drugs) [8].

An example of proarrhythmia due to treatment that included flecainide was recently published [6]. The authors reported on a 46-year-old woman with ventricular tachycardia and ventricular fibrillation after starting antiarrhythmic drug therapy with flecainide. The flecainide acetate plasma levels were always in the normal range. A successful therapeutic intervention was induced with two i.v. applications of 1000 mg magnesium glutamate. A persistent suppression of ventricular rhythm disturbance was accomplished by continuous i.v. application of 4 mg magnesium glutamate/min.

Despite ample criticism concerning the design of CAST and conclusions based on the study [1, 2, 5, 11] it seems obvious that flecainide and encainide are contraindicated in patients who meet the criteria of CAST, namely asymptomatic premature ventricular contractions and/or asymptomatic nonsustained ventricu-

Table 1. Antiarrhythmic therapy with flecainide

Recommended indications for flecainide
- Paroxysmal supraventricular tachycardias, including atrioventricular nodal reentrant tachycardia, atrioventricular reentrant tachycardia and other supraventricular tachycardias of unspecified mechanism
- Paroxysmal atrial fibrillation/flutter
- Symptomatic sustained ventricular tachycardia
- Premature ventricular contractions and/or nonsustained ventricular tachycardia causing disabling symptoms

Recommended contraindications for flecainide (CAST patients)
- Asymptomatic premature ventricular contractions and/or asymptomatic nonsustained ventricular tachycardia in patients with history of myocardial infarction

Recommendations for initiation of treatment with oral flecainide
- For patients with paroxysmal supraventricular arrhythmias, oral flecainide therapy may be started on an outpatient basis
- For patients with symptomatic sustained ventricular tachycardia, oral flecainide therapy should be started in the hospital
- For patients with premature ventricular contractions and/or nonsustained ventricular tachycardia causing disabling symptoms, a decision regarding outpatient or inpatient initiation of oral flecainide therapy must be based upon the physician's assessment of the individual patient

lar tachycardia in patients with a history of myocardial infarction and depressed left ventricular function. However there are different views between the decisions of national and international regulatory health authorities and the cardiologist's judgement (Table 1).

In the light of new data emerging from CAST results, the Cardiorenal Drugs Advisory Committee of the FDA reviewed CAST and released relevant recommendations on October 5 and 6, 1989:

1. Whether life-threatening arrhythmias – in addition to ventricular tachycardia – are an indication for flecainide should remain in the judgement of the physician.
2. The indication for other 1c antiarrhythmic substances like propafenone and indecainide should also be restricted to life-threatening ventricular arrhythmias.
3. 1a und 1b antiarrhythmic drugs should not be used in asymptomatic postmyocardial infarction patients, which was the population studied in CAST.
4. The labelling of all 1a and 1b antiarrhythmic drugs should include the statement that "no benefit with respect to mortality has been shown for any antiarrhythmic drug."
5. Flecainide should be approved for use in patients with symptomatic supraventricular arrhythmias without structural heart disease. The drug should be reserved for use in patients who present with debilitating symptoms.

In summary, the study has general implications indeed for the management of patients with arrhythmias. It has highlighted the potential harm associated with these agents. CAST has demonstrated a fact that we have actually known all along; the side effects of antiarrhythmic agents are significant, and sometimes even fatal [3]. As a result of the trial nonpharmacological treatment for arrhythmias (such as antitachycardia pacemakers, implantable cardioverter/defibrillators, catheterablation and heart transplantation) seem likely to be considered more readily, though these strategies, too, carry some risk. As for the use of flecainide in the management of ventricular tachycardia, it can be suggested that flecainide (and encainide) should not be firstline therapy. However, it should continue to be given when other drugs have failed in the treatment of these life-threatening arrhythmias. Probably it is appropriate to say that more patients are now likely to suffer because therapy with flecainide is withheld than will suffer because of the already well-recognized arrhythmogenic potential of the drug [7].

In conclusion, as far as the question concerns whether there has been a change in antiarrhythmic approach after CAST, the answer is yes! The practical implication for the clinician is that – based on CAST – neither flecainide nor encainide should be used in patients with asymptomatic ventricular premature beats after myocardial infarction (and depressed LV function); however, additional placebo-controlled mortality trials among patients who are at high risk for sudden death are warranted. CAST will provide the impetus to investigate the electrophysiology of sudden cardiac death and the mechanisms of action and proarrhythmic effects of antiarrhythmic drugs.

The paper by S. Saksena, Newark, N.J., was entitled "Nonpharmacologic Therapy for Malignant Ventricular Tachyarrhythmias in Patients with Congestive Heart Failure." The author came to the conclusion that an implantable cardioverter/defibrillator will provide a serious therapeutic option for patients with congestive heart failure and sustained ventricular tachycardia or ventricular fibrillation. Implantation of endocardial lead systems will reduce implant morbidity and mortality to acceptable levels. Use of multiprogrammable devices and the availability of multiple electrical therapies will provide for treatment of both bradycardias and tachycardias in these patients. This should permit this nonpharmacologic approach to be used in conjunction with aggressive management techniques for congestive heart failure. Implant of epicardial lead system may be restricted in the future to patients undergoing major cardiac surgical procedures for their congestive heart failure. Implantable cardioverter/defibrillator therapy would be applicable to patients with paroxysmal ventricular tachycardia for ventricular fibrillation, irrespective of rate morphology or underlying heart disease. It can be expected to be used in conjunction with antiarrhythmic drug therapy or ablation techniques. Implantable cardioverter/defibrillator therapy will also be available as alternative therapy for patients who are only partially or inadequately controlled by drug or ablation therapy. These nonpharmacologic approaches for the treatment of sustained ventricular tachyarrhythmias will offer an important alternative to current pharmacologic approaches, particularly in patients with significant left ventricular dysfunction and congestive heart failure (Saksena, this volume).

Thus, chronic recurrent ventricular tachycardia (VT) can be terminated reproducibly by electrotherapeutic tools such as programmed endocardial right ventricular stimulation or an implantable cardioverter/defribrillator. However, antitachycardia pacing is associated with a possible acceleration of VT, while frequent occurrence of VT and discomfort of the patient can limit treatment with an implantable cardioverter/defibrillator.

Recently, the combined use of antitachycardia pacing (Tachylog pacemaker; Siemens-Elema) and AICD (automatic implantable cardioverter/defibrillator, Cardiac Pacemakers Inc.) was evaluated in 6 of 40 patients (aged 50 to 70 years, mean 60.1 ± 7.7) in whom AICD had been implanted because of VT, which could be terminated by temporary overdrive pacing. With the interactive mode of the Tachylog, termination of VT by the pacemaker as well as by the AICD was assessed after implantation.

In the automatic mode, the Tachylog functioned as a bipolar ventricular inhibited (VVI) device with antitachycardia burst stimulation: 2–5 stimuli, interval 260–300 ms, 1–2 interventions. During follow-up of 47 ± 24 months, the Tachylog terminated VT reliably 50–505 times per patient. When burst stimulation accelerated VT, termination was achieved by AICD discharge. Thus, drug-resistant VT can be terminated by antitachycardia pacing, avoiding patient discomfort. In case of acceleration, VT can be controlled by the AICD. A universal pacemaker should combine antibradycardia and antitachycardia pacing with back-up cardioversion/defibrillation mode [4].

Conclusion

Primary treatment of cardiac arrhythmias tries to influence the underlying heart disease (Fig. 1). Symptomatic therapy is subdivided into drug therapy, electrotherapeutic tools (e.g., antitachycardia pacemaker, implantable cardioverter/

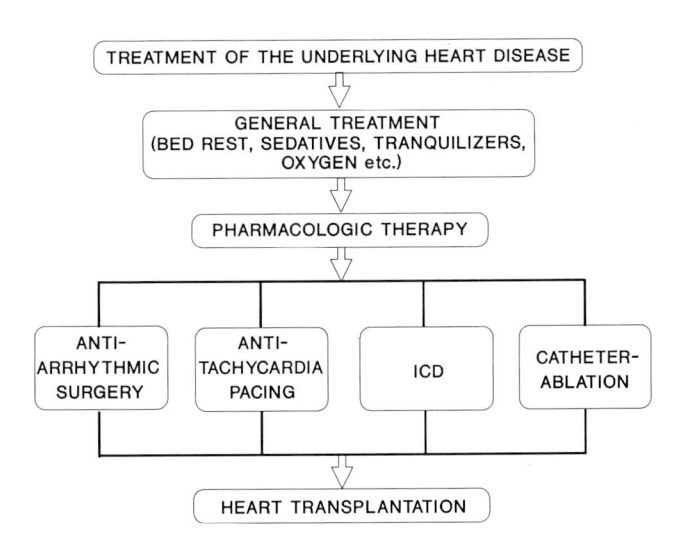

Fig. 1. Management of cardiac arrhythmias in congestive heart failure. *ICD* = implantable cardioverter/defibrillator

defibrillator), fulguration (ablation), and antiarrhythmic surgery and heart transplantation.

It is readily conceivable that the possibilities of antiarrhythmic therapy in tachyarrhythmias today are more effective, but at the same time more complicated than they were a few years ago. This is equally true for the indication of therapy in general, for the decision to apply a particular therapeutic measure, and for the control of antiarrhythmic treatment itself, especially in congestive heart failure.

In view of the progress in antiarrhythmic therapy, it seems likely to further reduce the number of drug resistant cardiac arrhythmias in patients who also have congestive heart failure.

Nevertheless, some important questions remain to be answered:

Is long-term antiarrhythmic therapy of asymptomatic ventricular arrhythmias in congestive heart failure reasonable or even necessary?
Does such treatment of ventricular arrhythmias suppress or limit sudden cardiac death following myocardial infarction when ventricular dysfunction is present?
Can the reduction of the re-infarction incidence by beta-receptor blocking agents be explained as an antiarrhythmic effect?
Is the arrhythmia itself or the underlying cardiac disease with decreased ventricular function decisive for the clinical symptoms or progression and prognosis?
Do new, more effective antiarrhythmic drugs make surgical treatment of cardiac arrhythmias largely dispensable?
Does the implantable cardioverter/defibrillator have a future in the large number of patients with a history of congestive heart failure and life-threatening arrhythmias?

The answers to these and other questions can only be given by controlled, prospective long-term studies. In view of the frequently well-tolerated arrhythmias and the considerable rate of cardiac and extracardiac side effects associated with antiarrhythmic interventions, a critical consideration of the individual case still appears urgently required prior to induction of any antiarrhythmic therapy.

References

1. Anonymous (1989) Flecainide and CAST. Lancet II:481–482
2. Garratt C, Ward DE, Camm AJ (1989) Lessons from the cardiac arrhythmia suppression trial. Br Med J 299:805–806
3. Gottlieb SS (1979) The use of antiarrhythmic agents in heart failure: implications of CAST. Am Heart J 118:1074–1077
4. Lüderitz B, Manz M (1989) Role of antitachycardia devices in the treatment of ventricular tachyarrhythmias. Am J Cardiol 64:75J–78J
5. Lüderitz B (1990) Did the antiarrhythmic approach change after CAST? New Trends Arrhyt VI:235–239
6. Mletzko R, Jung W, Manz M, Kamradt T, Vogel F, Lüderitz B (1989) Proarrhythmic effect of flecainide-therapy with magnesium i.v. Z Kardiol 78:602–606
7. Morgan J (1989) The fall of flecainide. Cardiol Pract 11–12
8. Ruskin JN (1989) The Cardiac Arrhythmia Suppression Trial (CAST). N Engl J Med 321:386–388

9. The Cardiac Arrhythmia Pilot Study (CAPS) investigators (1988) Effects of encainide, flecainide, imipramine and moricizine on ventricular arrhythmias during the year after acute myocardial infarction: the CAPS. Am J Cardiol 61:501–509
10. The Cardiac Arrhythmia Suppression Trial (CAST) investigators (1989) Preliminary report: effect of encainide and flecainide on mortality in a randomized trial of arrhythmia suppression after myocardial infarction. N Engl J Med 321:406–412
11. Ward D, Garratt C, Camm AJ (1989) Cardiac arrhythmia suppression trial and flecainide. Lancet I:1267–1268

When to Treat Arrhythmias in Heart Failure?

A. P. M. Gorgels, P. Brugada, and H. J. J. Wellens

Introduction

Clinical medicine is characterized by a continuous process of decision making based on optimal diagnostic information leading to the most appropriate therapeutic approach. Very important in this process is individualization of the approach. Every patient presents with his or her particular manifestation of a disease, and in every case the clinician has to unravel its specific features. Only in this way is he able to offer the patient optimal benefit from the many therapeutic possibilities available today with the least discomfort or risk.

These general comments hold especially when discussing the treatment of arrhythmias occurring in the setting of heart failure. Optimal treatment of arrhythmias in the failing heart is dependent on many factors which have to be considered in order to adjust the different treatment modalities to the specific problem of the patient.

Pathophysiological Aspects of Arrhythmias and Heart Failure

In Fig. 1 the factors playing a role in the occurrence of an arrhythmia are schematically presented. Electrical instability, ischemia, and hemodynamic dysfunction are major contributing factors leading to initiation or perpetuation of an arrhythmia. The diagram emphasizes that the different pathophysiological disorders have both static and dynamic components, and that their interplay promotes the occurrence of an arrhythmia. On the other hand, an arrhythmia itself may induce further ischemia or hemodynamic dysfunction, thus creating a vicious circle.

Arrhythmias may be the cause of heart failure especially when they are long-lasting or incessant, a syndrome which is called tachycardiomyopathy [1–5]. On the other hand, there are several ways by which hemodynamic dysfunction facilitates the occurrence of arrhythmias. It may lead to volume overload of the ventricles and subsequent stretching of myocardial tissue. It has been shown that stretch on Purkinje's fibers cause them to depolarize [6] resulting in slow conduction favoring the occurrence of reentry [7]. Depolarized Purkinje's fibers may exhibit abnormal automaticity and triggered activity [6]. Heart failure may also lead to activation of the sympathetic nervous system possibly causing increased

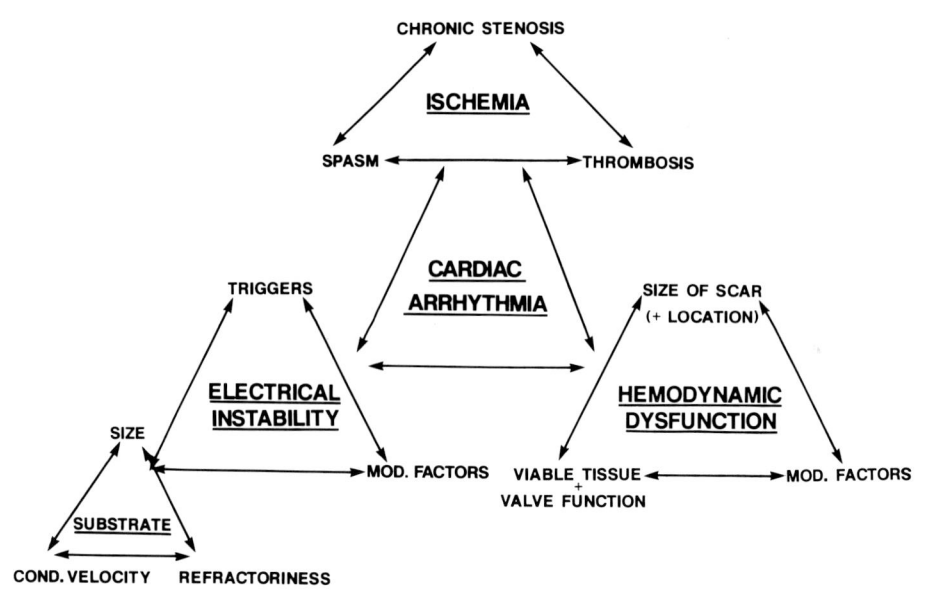

Fig. 1. Model showing the factors that play a role in cardiac arrhythmias. The basic triangle consists of electrical instability, hemodynamic dysfunction, and ischemia. Each of these three cornerstones has static and dynamic components. Modulating factors include the autonomic nervous system, electrolytes, hormones (renin-angiotensine system) and drugs

ventricular irritability. Activation of the sympathetic nervous system and the renin-angiotensin system may also induce hypokalemia, particularly in the presence of diuretic drugs [8]. Hypokalemia and hypomagnesemia may lead to torsade de pointes, especially when combined with class I antiarrhythmic drugs. Digitalis intoxication, which is facilitated by electrolyte disturbances may cause arrhythmias and conduction disturbances at different levels in the heart [9–10].

As already alluded to, an important aspect in relation to the treatment of arrhythmias in patients with heart failure is that electrical instability, ischemia, and hemodynamic dysfunction each have components with a more dynamic or static behavior. Considering ischemia, for instance, which is a major cause of arrhythmias [11, 12], its degree in a given patient is related to the severity of the fixed stenosis in the coronary artery, but also to dynamic factors such as spasm and thrombogenicity. Other static factors are scar tissue of a myocardial infarction, the substrate for reentry, or the degree of valve dysfunction in a patient with valvular heart disease. Static factors are difficult to manipulate pharmacologically and frequently need invasive treatment approaches, whereas dynamic factors such as spasm, thrombosis, influences of the autonomic nervous system, and properties of a reentry circuit are accessible to drug treatment.

A final consideration is the different and frequently opposite effect of drugs on the three above-mentioned pathophysiological components. For example, drugs which diminish ischemia, such as beta-blocking agents, impair pump function, or drugs improving pump function may increase electrical instability, such as phosphodiesterase inhibitors [13]. Class I antiarrhythmic drugs may suppress reentrant arrhythmias but concomitantly induce QT-prolongation leading to Torsade de Pointes.

As has been mentioned above, it is crucial for appropriate management that the importance of these different factors is determined in the individual patient – indicating that a good arrhythmologist above all needs to be a good clinician.

When to Treat Arrhythmias in Heart Failure?

To discuss the problem of which arrhythmias occurring in patients with heart failure require treatment, three questions must be answered: (a) Does the arrhythma cause heart failure? (b) Does the arrhythmia present symptoms? (c) Does the arrhythmia worsen prognosis?

Does the Arrhythmia Cause Heart Failure?

In tachycardia-related cardiomyopathy congestive heart failure is completely or largely secondary to tachycardia [1–5]. Such a tachycardia may be of supraventricular or ventricular origin. In most instances these tachycardias have an incessant nature. Because of the persistingly high rate biventricular failure develops gradually and may dominate the clinical picture. It is not unusual that the real cause of events is not understood, and that tachycardia is seen as secondary to heart failure in these patients instead of the reverse: heart failure because of the persistent arrhythmia. Subsequently attention is given only to treatment of heart failure. This may occur especially in supraventricular tachycardias such as atrial fibrillation with high ventricular rates, atrial flutter, atrial tachycardia, and the incessant form of tachycardias using a slowly retrogradely conducting accessory pathway [14]. The appropriate approach is immediate termination and prevention of recurrences. Termination is especially effective when forms of treatment without negative inotropic effects are used. Atrial fibrillation may respond well to electrical cardioversion, but when these arrhythmias are recurrent or persistent with high ventricular rates, they must be controlled by ablating the atrioventricular conduction system [4]. In atrial tachycardia and flutter overdrive stimulation is frequently effective. The incessant form of circus-movement tachycardia in which a slowly conducting retrograde accessory pathway (Fig. 2) is incorporated in the tachycardia circuit is preferably treated by surgical ablation [5] of the accessory pathway [15, 16] because antiarrhythmic drug therapy usually fails to suppress the arrhythmia. After sinus rhythm has been restored, heart failure subsides within a few weeks, and heart size and ventricular wall motion return to normal (Fig. 3).

Occasionally, ventricular tachycardia (VT) may occur in a persistent or incessant form leading to severe pump failure. Again, restoration of sinus rhythm frequently results in marked improvement of pump function. Unfortunately, class I drugs may be hazardous by interfering with pump function and may even let the tachycardia persist because of their proarrhythmic potential [17, 18].

When to Treat Arrhythmias in Heart Failure? 103

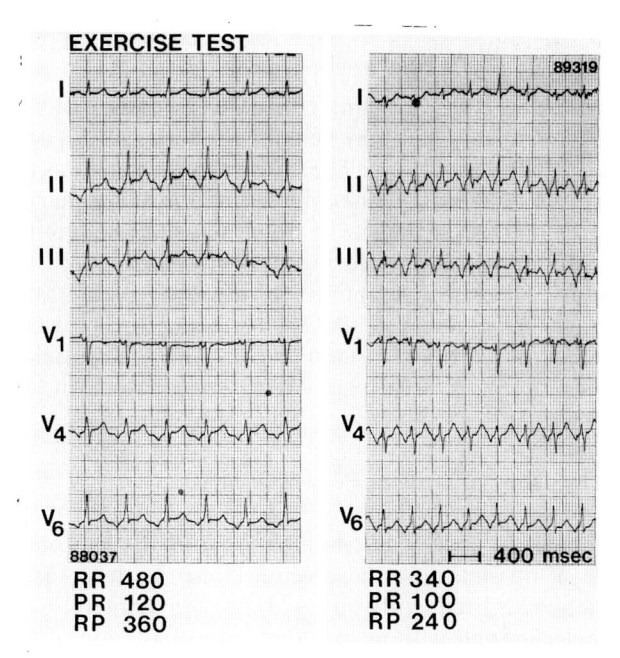

Fig. 2. Example of an incessant circus-movement tachycardia using a slowly retrogradely conducting pathway. The PR interval is shorter than the RP interval. The P-waves are negative in leads II, III, and AVF and in the left precordial leads. *Right panel*, during exercise the ventricular rate accelerates with shortening of both PR and RP intervals

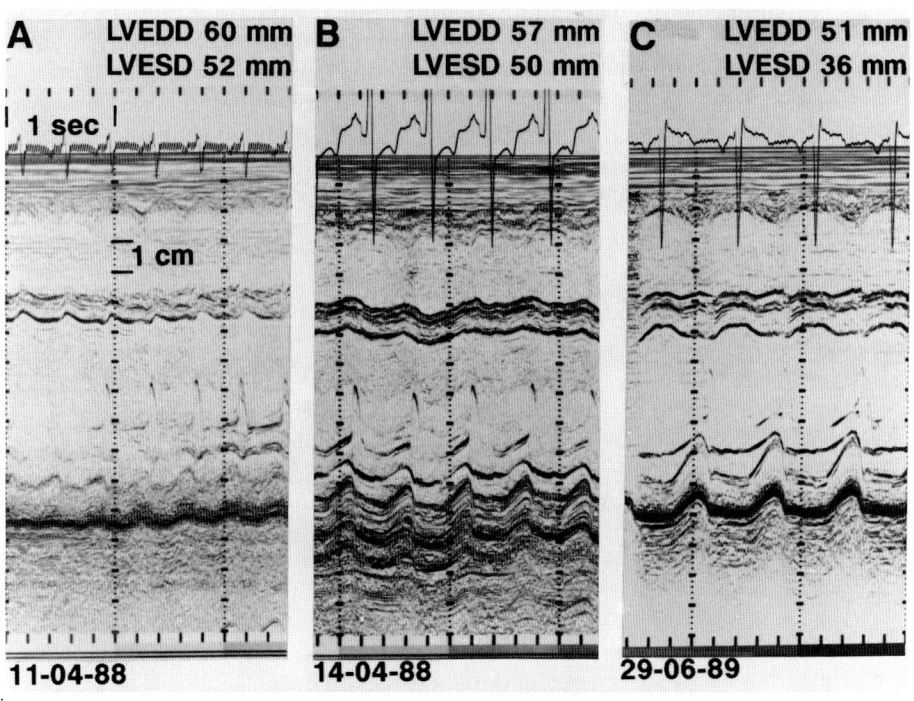

RR 480
PR 120
RP 360

RR 340
PR 100
RP 240

Fig. 3. M-mode echocardiographic recording of the left ventricle during and after termination of incessant circus-movement tachycardia (**A**), directly after (**B**), and 14 months after surgical ablation (**C**) of the slowly retrogradely conducting accessory pathway. Note the slight (**B**) and marked (**C**) improvement of left ventricular function, as assessed by a decrease in end-diastolic and end-systolic diameter. (Courtesy of E. Cheriex)

Recently, new methods have become available to terminate VT with nonpharmacological means. Tachycardia can be terminated surgically by endocardial resection [19], encircling endocardial ventriculotomy [20], or cryoablation [21]. Nonsurgically this may be done by electrical [22] or chemical ablation [23] of the arrhythmogenic area. The latter technique ablates the site of origin of the tachycardia by injecting ethanol in a peripheral coronary branch that supplies the VT area [23]. After the site of origin has been determined by catheter mapping, the coronary branch perfusing this area is visualized through selective catheterization. Thereafter temporary termination of VT is attempted by injecting cold saline to demonstrate that the correct coronary artery has been catheterized. This is followed by pure ethanol injection into the vessel to definitely terminate VT by destroying the area from which it originates. An example is given in Fig. 4.

Does the Arrhythmia Present Symptoms?

Goals of clinical medicine are to (a) relieve symptoms, (b) improve prognosis, and (c) if possible cure the disease. Unfortunately, the latter two cannot always be achieved. Frequently our goals must be limited to alleviation of symptoms without cure and without prolongation of the life of the patient. Arrhythmias can cause symptoms such as palpitations, dizziness, or collapse. Interestingly, however, many patients do not notice their arrhythmias and are completely asymptomatic. We have studied in a series of 83 patients the factors which determine a sensation of palpitations during sustained tachycardias (unpublished observations). The importance of the following factors were analyzed (Table 1): age, sex, arrhythmia variables (rate, site of origin, and regularity of the tachycardia),

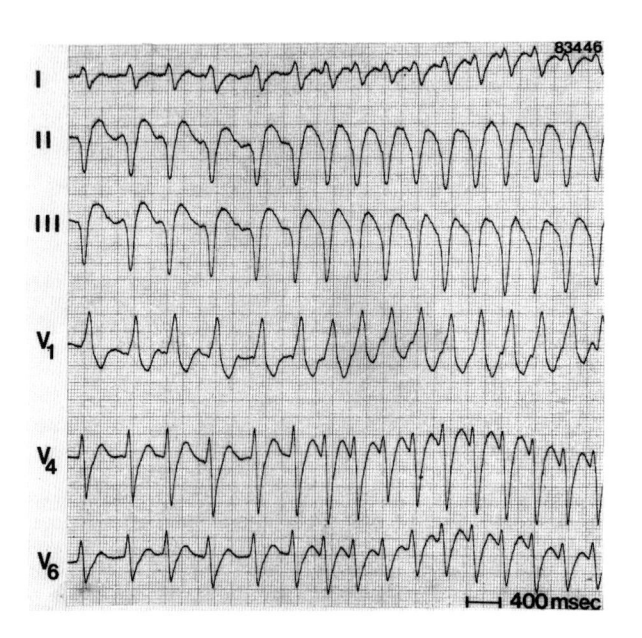

Fig. 4. Spontaneous acceleration of a ventricular tachycardia possibly based upon a change from one to two circulating impulses within one circuit during injection of class I antiarrhythmic drug. Simultaneous recording of six surface ECG leads. Note identical QRS configuration before and during acceleration

Table 1. Factors determining recognition of palpitations during sustained tachycardia in 83 patients

	Palpitations	No palpitations	P
No. of patients	57	26	
Age (years)	53 ± 20	69 ± 8	<0.001
Men/Women	31/27	21/4	<0.01
Rate/min	163 ± 40	157 ± 61	NS
SVT/VT	48/9	13/13	<0.01
Old infarct	12	8	NS
LVEDD	54 ± 10	54 ± 9	NS
FS	0.28 ± 0.12	0.26 ± 0.13	NS
CT ratio	0.52 ± 0.10	0.50 ± 0.09	NS
LVEF	47 ± 9	36 ± 7	<0.01

SVT, Supraventricular tachycardia (all forms); VT, ventricular tachycardia; LVEDD, left ventricular end-diastolic dimension, as measured by M-mode echocardiography; FS, fractional shortening, as measured echocardiographically; CT, cardiothoracic ratio on chest ray; LVEF, left ventricular ejection fraction.

factors related to pump function (systolic and diastolic diameter of the left ventricle, ejection fraction), and heart size (chest X ray). Awareness of tachycardia was related to age, sex, and origin of the arrhythmia. Tachycardias were less frequently experienced at older age, in women, and in ventricular rather than supraventricular tachycardias.

When arrhythmias are asymptomatic, it is questionable whether they should be treated. This holds especially when prognosis is not impaired by the arrhythmia. This is frequently the case when pump function is intact, and no ischemia is present. Examples are chronic atrial fibrillation with acceptable ventricular rates, especially in the older population, nonsustained ventricular arrhythmias occurring without overt heart disease [24–27], and simple forms of ventricular arrhythmias after a myocardial infarction, single or pairs of ventricular premature depolarization, VPD, in the setting of a preserved left ventricular ejection fraction [28]. Antiarrhythmic drug treatment is also frequently not needed in tachycardia, which although symptomatic are benign and occur infrequently. Examples are circus-movement tachycardias using an accessory pathway or AV nodal tachycardias, which not infrequently can be terminated by having the patient perform a vagal maneuver. Antiarrhythmic drug treatment has not only side effects which may interfere with quality of life but possibly also, as mentioned above, proarrhythmic effects. Drugs which slow conduction velocity may change a nonsustained tachycardia into a sustained one and may even accelerate a sustained tachycardia.

Recently a new mechanism has been described explaining sudden acceleration of sustained VT [29]. This mechanism has been named double-wave reentry and has been observed in Langendorf perfused rings of anisotropic rabbit epicardium. In these preparations tachycardia could be accelerated by pacing by inducing two instead of one circulating impulses within the same circuit. It was also possible to induce double-wave reentry after administration of class I drugs in experiments in which only single-wave reentry was obtained during control conditions. Figure 5 shows an example of a clinical VT acceleration following administration of a class I drug. Although other mechanisms may be involved it is possible that double-wave reentry is the underlying mechanism of the acceleration.

Does the Arrhythmia Worsen Prognosis?

Another important consideration as to whether arrhythmias should be treated is the prognostic significance of an arrhythmia. The arrhythmia may have no prognostic meaning, outcome being mainly determined by the underlying cardiac disease. Another possibility is that an arrhythmia is a predictor but not the cause of poor outcome, that is, it increases the chance for nonsudden death. Thirdly, the arrhythmia may be the cause of a bad prognosis, predicting an increased risk for sudden cardiac death.

Prognosis of Ventricular Tachycardia Depends on Underlying Etiology

It has been well demonstrated that prognosis in patients with sustained VT is dependent on the underlying etiology [24–27, 30–33]. Prognosis is known to be excellent in idiopathic VT and in right ventricular dysplasia. In a group of 52 patients without overt cardiac disease presenting with sustained or nonsustained VT followed up at our institution [27] no cardiac death was documented during a mean follow-up of 8 years. In contrast, the prognosis in patients with VT occurring after myocardial infarction or in the setting of nonischemic dilated cardiomyopathy prognosis is worse. Risk stratification in relation to prognosis has been performed in 200 patients with VT or ventricular fibrillation after the acute phase of myocardial infarction [32]. Four variables were found to be predictive for an increased risk for sudden or nonsudden death during a mean follow-up of 2 years: (a) cardiac arrest at the time of the first spontaneous episode of arrhythmia; (b) dyspnea functional class III according to the New York Heart association; (c) early occurrence of VT after myocardial infarction (after 3 days and within 2 months); (d) the presence of multiple myocardial infarctions.

Patients with none or one variable had an incidence of sudden death of 2.8% and an incidence of 4.2% of nonsudden cardiac death (Figs. 5, 6) while patients with more than two variables had a 13.5% and 20.3% incidence, respectively, of sudden and nonsudden cardiac death. The strongest predictor of sudden death was the occurrence of cardiac arrest during the first spontaneous episode of ventricular arrhythmia. The strongest predictor of nonsudden death was the functional class of the patient.

These findings stress the importance of the hemodynamic effect of the arrhythmia and the degree of heart failure outside the tachycardia episodes in deciding whether an arrhythmia should be treated.

When to Treat Arrhythmias in Heart Failure?

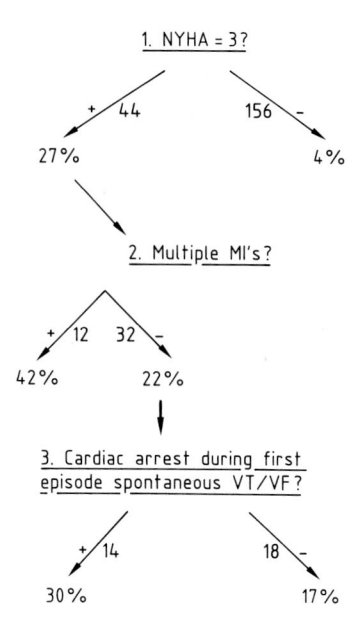

```
                                    1. NYHA = 3?
                                   /            \
                              +  / 44         156 \  -
                             27%                    4%
                               \
                                \
                                 2. Multiple MI's?
                                /               \
                           + / 12              32 \ -
                          42%                      22%
                                                    ↓
                                         3. Cardiac arrest during first
                                         episode spontaneous VT/VF?
                                                /        \
                                           + / 14       18 \ -
                                          30%               17%
```

Fig. 5. Risk of nonsudden death in 200 patients using four clinical parameters (see text) in ventricular tachycardia (*VT*) or ventricular fibrillation (*VF*) after myocardial infarction (*MI*). Risk at 2 years was 9%

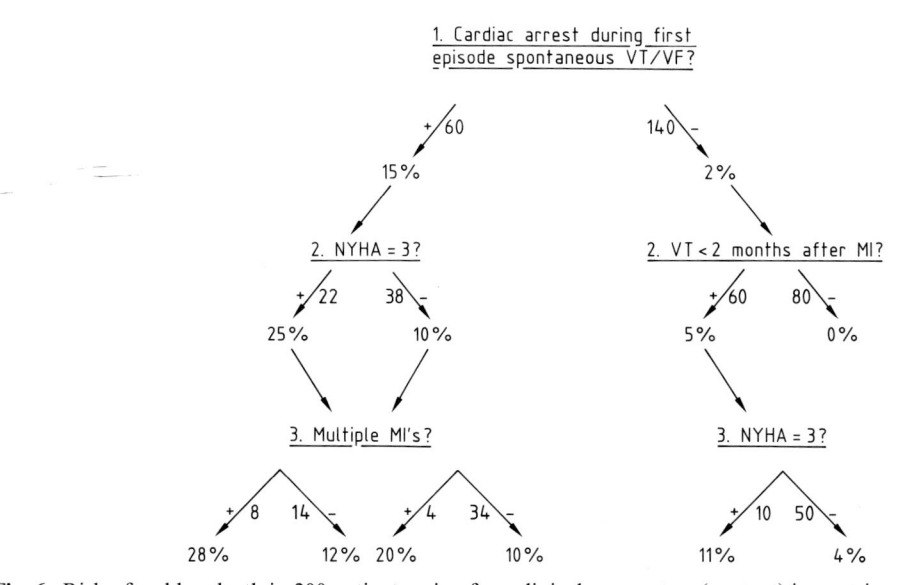

```
                           1. Cardiac arrest during first
                           episode spontaneous VT/VF?
                          /                              \
                     + / 60                             140 \ -
                     15%                                     2%
                      /                                       \
            2. NYHA = 3?                            2. VT < 2 months after MI?
           /           \                            /                      \
       + / 22        38 \ -                    + / 60                    80 \ -
       25%              10%                    5%                           0%
         \              /                       \
          \            /                         \
           3. Multiple MI's?                      3. NYHA = 3?
          /     \    /    \                      /          \
       +/ 8  14 \-  +/ 4  34 \-                +/ 10      50 \-
       28%   12%   20%    10%                  11%           4%
```

Fig. 6. Risk of sudden death in 200 patients using four clinical parameters (see text) in ventricular tachycardia (*VT*) or ventricular fibrillation (*VF*) after myocardial infarction (*MI*). Risk at 2 years was 6%

Four clinical situations can be recognized in relation to prognosis and subsequent need for treatment.

1. Arrhythmias may occur without interfering with prognosis. Examples are circus-movement tachycardia in the Wolff-Parkinson-White syndrome, idiopathic VT, and VT in right ventricular dysplasia. In these instances antiarrhythmic drug therapy is indicated only to prevent recurrences but not to prolong life. The same holds for sustained VT occurring after myocardial infarction. In our series we found that when tachycardia is hemodynamically well tolerated, and outside the tachycardia no or only mild signs of heart failure are present, the 2-year prognosis is excellent [32]. Also in this group of patients, antiarrhythmic drug therapy is needed only to prevent recurrences. In order to prevent negative inotropic and proarrhythmic effects it may even be considered to avoid antiarrhythmic drug therapy when the incidence of arrhythmia attacks is low.

2. A clear indication for antiarrhythmic drug therapy in relation to prognosis is present when VT secondary to myocardial infarction is hemodynamically poorly tolerated. Patients surviving the initial episode were found to have a fivefold increased risk of dying suddenly within the next 2 years. When outside the VT episode no or only mild signs of heart failure are present, antiarrhythmic drugs can be given safely. Although no randomized placebo-controlled studies have been conducted to assess the benefit of antiarrhythmic drugs in these patients, it is generally accepted to prescribe antiarrhythmic drug therapy.

3. More complicated is the situation when both the arrhythmia is poorly tolerated, and the patient is in heart failure outside the tachycardia episode. Here the 2-years risk for dying suddenly increases about tenfold (from 2% to 20%). Therefore optimal antiarrhythmic therapy is indicated preferably with the least negative effect on pump function. Because of the poor prognosis more aggressive options such as amiodarone, electrical or ethanol ablation, or surgical resection of the site of origin must be considered.

4. Most controversy exists in relation to asymptomatic ventricular arrhythmias occurring in patients with heart failure. It has been shown that in 80% of these cases heart failure occurs in the setting of coronary artery disease and in 10%–15% because of cardiomyopathy [34]. These arrhythmias are often asymptomatic because they are nonsustained. Ambulatory electrocardiographic monitoring [34, 35] has shown in several studies a prevalence of single VPD between 91% and 100%, complex VPD between 36% and 95%, and nonsustained VT between 23% and 60%. Sudden unexpected mortality varied in the different studies from 30% to 45% of total number of deaths during 1-year follow-up. Because of the high prevalence of sudden death in patients with heart failure, there is growing interest in the role of ventricular arrhythmias in relation to prognosis and the possible value of antiarrhythmic treatment.

There is convincing evidence that complex ventricular arrhythmias are independent predictors for sudden and non-sudden cardiac death in patients with pump failure [34, 35]. The question whether suppression of these arrhythmias by antiarrhythmic drug therapy will improve prognosis is presently unanswered. The results of the CAST study [36] emphasize some of the problems with antiarrhythmic drug therapy. Flecainide and encainide (after having shown to be able to suppress ventricular ectopic activity) resulted in a higher death rate than in patients receiving placebo. The results of this and other ongoing trials studying the effect of other antiarrhythmic drugs must be awaited before more definite conclusions can be drawn.

In conclusion, in selecting modes of treatment all factors contributing to the occurrence of an arrhythmia must be taken into account. Treatment of arrhythmias in heart failure is indicated when the arrhythmia is causing heart failure, is presenting sufficiently severe symptoms, or when the arrhythmia impairs prognosis. In selecting antiarrhythmic drugs, benefit should be weighed against risk of side effects, proarrhythmic effects, and the increased risk of heart failure.

References

1. Coleman HN, Taylor RR, Pool PE, Whipple GH, Covell JN, Ross JR, Braunwald E (1971) Congestive heart failure following chronic tachycardia. Am Heart J 81:750–798
2. Damiano JR, Tripp HF, Small KW, Asano T, Jones RH, Lowe IE (1985) The functional consequences of prolonged supraventricular tachycardia. J Am Coll Cardiol 5:541
3. Packer DL, Bardy GH, Worley SJ, Smith MS, Cobb FR, Coleman E, Gallagher JJ, German LD (1986) Tachycardia induced cardiomyopathy: a reversible form of left ventricular dysfunction. Am J Cardiol 57:563–570
4. Lemery R, Brugada P, Cheriex E, Wellens HJJ (1987) Reversibility of tachycardia-induced left ventricular dysfunction after closed-chest catheter ablation of the atrioventricular junction for intractable atrial fibrillation. Am J Cardiol 60:1406–1408
5. Cruz FES, Brugada P, Smeets JLRM, Atie J, Duque M, Guang Fei S, Oyarzun R, Peres AK, Cheriex EC, Penn OCKM, Wellens HJJ (1990) Reversibility of tachycardia-induced cardiomyopathy after surgical cure of incessant supraventricular tachycardia. Eur Heart J 10:226 (abstract)
6. Bigger JT Jr (1973) Electrical properties of cardiac muscle and possible causes of cardiac arrhythmias. In: Dreifus LS, Likoff (eds) Cardiac arrhythmias. Grune and Stratton, New York, p 13
7. Cranefield PF, Klein HO, Hoffman BF (1971) Conduction on the cardiac impulse. I. Delay, block and one-way block in depressed Purkinje fibers. Circ Res 28:199–204
8. Cohn JN, Levine TB, Olivari MT, Garberg V, Lura D, Francis GS, Simon A, Rector T (1984) Plasma norepinephrine as a guide to prognosis in patients with chronic congestive heart failure. N Engl J Med 311:819
9. Wellens HJJ (1976) The electrocardiogram in digitalis intoxication. In: Yu PN, Goodwin JF (eds) Progress in cardiology. Lea and Febiger, Philadelphia, pp 271–290
10. Vanagt EJ, Wellens HJJ (1981) The electrocardiogram digitalis intoxication. In: Wellens HJ, Kulbertus HE (eds) What's new in electrocardiography? Nyhoff, The Hague, pp 315–343
11. Wit AL, Bigger JT Jr (1975) Possible electrophysiological mechanisms for lethal arrhythmias accompanying myocardial ischemia and infarction. Circulation 52 Suppl III:III-96
12. Janse MJ (1987) Arrhythmias during acute ischemia in experimental models. In: Brugada P, Wellens HJ (eds) Cardiac arrhythmias: where do we go from here? Futura, Mount Kisco, pp 105–128
13. Anderson JL, Askins JC, Gilbert EM, Menlove RL, Lutz JR (1986) Occurrence of ventricular arrhythmias in patients receiving acute and chronic infusions of Milrinone. Am Heart J 111:466–474
14. Coumel P, Attuel P, Leclercq JF (1979) Permanent form of junctional reciprocating tachycardia: mechanism, clinical and therapeutic implications. In: Narulaos (ed) Cardiac arrhythmias. pp 347–363. William and Wilkins, Baltimore
15. Guiraudon JM, Klein GJ, Sharma AD, Jones DL, McLellan DG (1986) Surgical ablation of posterior septal accessory pathways in the Wolff-Parkinson-White syndrome by a closed heart technique. J Thorac Cardiovasc Surg 92:406–413

16. Sealy WC, Gallagher JJ (1980) The surgical approach to the septal area of the heart based on the experiences with forty-five patients with Kent bundles. J Thorac Cardiovasc Surg 79:542–551
17. Podrid PJ (1985) Aggravation of ventricular arrhythmias. A drug-induced complication. Drugs [Suppl 4] 33
18. Morganroth J, Anderson JL, Gentzkow GD (1986) Classification by type of ventricular arrhythmia predicts frequency of adverse cardiac events from flecainide. J Am Coll Cardiol 8:607
19. Josephson ME, Harken AH, Horowitz LN (1979) Endocardial excision: a new surgical technique for the treatment of recurrent ventricular tachycardia. Circulation 60:1430–1439
20. Guiraudon G, Fontaine J, Frank R, Escaude G, Etieveut P, Cabrol C (1978) Encircling endocardial ventriculotomy: a new surgical treatment for life-treatening ventricular tachycardias resistant to medical treatment following myocardial infarction. Ann Thorac Surg 26:438–444
21. Gallagher JJ, Anderson RW, Kasell JH, Rice JR, Pritchett ELC, Gault JH, Harrison LA, Wallace AG (1978) Cryoablation of drug-resistant ventricular tachycardia in a patient with a variant of scleroderma. Circulation 57:190
22. Hartzler GD (1983) Electrode catheter ablation of refractory focal ventricular tachycardia. J Am Cardiol 2:1107–1113
23. Brugada P, de Swart H, Smeets JLRM, Wellens HJJ (1989) Transcoronary chemical ablation of ventricular tachycardia. Circulation 79:475–482
24. Rahilli TG, Prystowski EN, Zipes DP, Naccarelli GV, Jackman WM, Heger JJ (1982) Clinical and electrophysiologic findings in patients with repetitive monomorphic ventricular tachycardia and otherwise normal electrocardiogram. Am J Cardiol 50:459–468
25. Buxton AE, Waxman HL, Marchlinski FE, Simson MB, Cassidy D, Josphson ME (1983) Right ventricular tachycardia: clinical and electrophysiological characteristics. Circulation 68:917–927
26. Deal BJ, Miller SM, Scagliotti D, Prechel D, Gallastegui JL, Hariman RJ (1986) Ventricular tachycardia in a young population without overt heart disease. Circulation 73:1111–1118
27. Lemery R, Brugada P, Della Bella P, Dugernier T, van den Dool A, Wellens HJJ (1989) Non-ischemic ventricular tachycardia. Clinical course and longterm follow up in patients without clinical overt heart disease. Circulation 79:990–999
28. Bigger TJ Jr, Fleiss JL, Kluger R, Miller JP, Rohnitzky LM, and the Multicenter Postinfarction Research Group (1984) The relationships among ventricular arrhythmias, left ventricular dysfunction and mortality in the 2 years after myocardial infarction. Circulation 69 (2):250–258
29. Brugada J, Boersma L, Brugada P, Havenith M, Wellens HJJ, Allessie M (1990) Double wave reentry as a mechanism of acceleration of ventricular tachycardia. (Circulation 1990, in press)
30. Franciosa JA, Wilen M, Ziesche S, Cohn JN (1983) Survival in men with severe chronic left ventricular failure due to either coronary heart disease or idiopathic dilated cardiomyopathy. Am J Cardiol 51:831–836
31. Holmes J, Kubo SH, Cody RJ, Kligfield P (1985) Arrhythmias in ischemic and non-ischemic dilated cardiomyopathy: prediction of mortality by ambulatory electrocardiography. Am J Cardiol 55:146–151
32. Brugada P, Talajic M, Smeets J, Mulleneers R, Wellens HJJ (1989) Risk stratification of patients with ventricular tachycardia or ventricular fibrillation after myocardial infarction. The value of the clinical history. Eur Heart J 10:747–752
33. Lemery R, Burgada P, Janssen J, Cheriex E, Dugernier T, Wellens HJJ (1989) Nonischemic sustained ventricular tachycardia: clinical outcome in 12 patients with arrhythmogenic right ventricular dysplasia. J Am Coll Cardiol 14:96–105
34. Bigger JT Jr (1987) Why patients with congestive heart failure die: arrhythmias and sudden cardiac death. Circulation 75 [Suppl IV]:IV-28
35. Massie BM, Conway M (1987) Survival of patients with congestive heart failure: post, present and future prospects. Circulation 75 [Suppl IV]:IV-11
36. Cardiac Arrhythmia Suppression Trial (CAST) (1989) Investigators preliminary report: effect of encainide and flecainide in mortality in a randomized trial of arrhythmic suppression after myocardial infarction. N Engl J Med 321:406–412

Antiarrhythmic Drugs in Heart Failure*

J. Brachmann, C. Schmitt, T. Beyer, B. Waldecker, T. Hilbel, M. Schweizer, and W. Kübler

It has been well established that death due to progressive heart failure is a major risk in patients with impaired cardiac function. However, the exact mechanism of death remains subject to controversy. While it is questionable whether the contribution of arrhythmias alone is responsible, it is a widely accepted fact that most patients finally die due to malignant arrhythmias [1–3]. Even more doubts arise around the problem of drug therapy directed to suppress arrhythmias in patients with impaired ventricular function. The results of the CAST trial, which are presented elsewhere in this book, have contributed to doubts about the value of nondiscriminative prophylactic therapy for spontaneous ectopy guided by Holter monitoring [4]. By contrast, the results of the consensus trial support the assumption that an improvement in left ventricular (LV) function by means of afterload reduction can improve the clinical outcome either by hemodynamic improvements alone or by direct antiarrhythmic action [5].

The experimental setup for analyzing the latter controversy more precisely consists of a conscious dog model which investigates the late postmyocardial infarction period 3–8 days after proximal ligation of the left anterior descending coronary artery. Details are described elsewhere [6]. The dogs were anesthetized with 30 mg/kg pentobarbital, and a left thoracotomy was performed. The left anterior descending coronary artery was exposed and a two-stage ligation was performed just distal of the septal artery. Epicardial composite electrodes were fixed to record potentials from the infarct zone and adjacent normal myocardium as well as to identify abnormal electrical activity potentially involved in reentrant arrhythmias. The thoracotomy was closed and the animals subsequently permitted to recover.

After 3–8 days, the animals were studied using surface electrogram and composite electrogram recordings obtained by means of programmed electrical stimulation. To demonstrate reproducibility, induction of sustained ventricular tachycardia was repeated unless external cardioversion had been employed to terminate the arrhythmia. Thereafter, the new angiotensin converting enzyme (ACE), inhibitor, cilazapril and its active metabolite cilazaprilate were administered intravenously at cumulative dosages of 1 mg/kg and 2 mg/kg on different days, respectively. This dosage was found to be hemodynamically effective in earlier experiments. The results are summarized in Fig. 1, and representative tracings are presented in Fig. 2. In these experiments, no significant alteration was observed

---

* This study was supported by the SFB 320 "Herzfunktion und ihre Regulation" and the Deutsche Forschungsgemeinschaft.

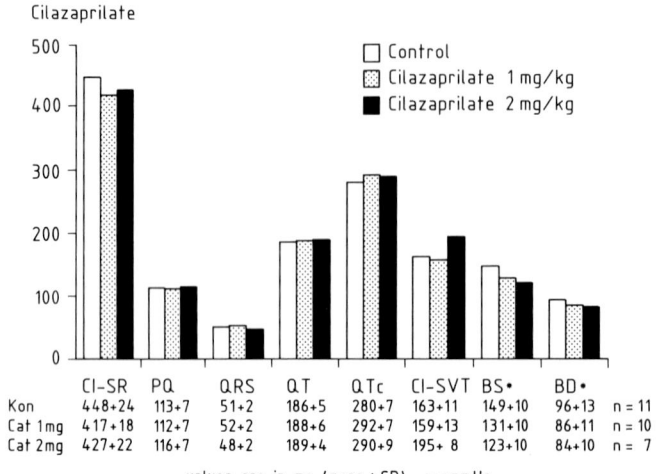

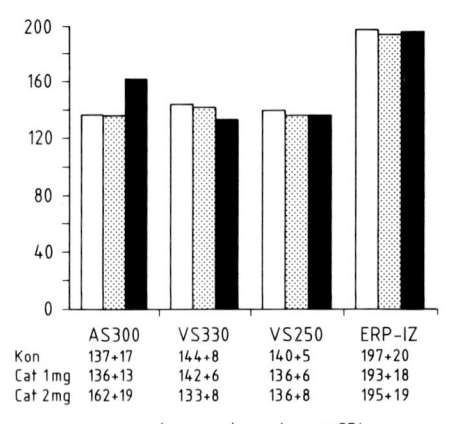

Fig. 1. Effects of the ACE inhibitor metabolite cilazaprilate 1 mg/kg and 2 mg/kg in 10 conscious dogs in the late postmyocardial infarction period. All values are presented as mean ± SD, differences between the increasing doses of cilazaprilate were analyzed by variance analysis. None of the electrophysiological parameters was significantly changed, while systolic and diastolic blood pressure significantly fell after administration of cilazaprilat. *Cl-SR*, cycle length of sinus rhythm; *PQ*, PQ interval; *QRS*, QRS interval; *QT*, QT interval; QT_c, QT_c interval corrected for sinus rate; *CL-SVT*, cycle length of the sustained ventricular tachycardia; *BS*, systolic blood pressure; *BP*, diastolic blood pressure; *AS 300*, atrial stimulation at 300 ms; *VS 330*, ventricular stimulation at 330 ms; *VS 250*, ventricular stimulation at 250 ms cycle length; ERP_{IZ}, effective refractory period of the infarct zone

in the electrophysiological parameters nor in the inducibility of ventricular tachyarrhythmias after administration of cilazapril and its active metabolite. Similar results were obtained in a dose-response curve recorded in action potentials from isolated preparations by means of standard microelectrode techniques. All parameters, including resting potential, action potential amplitude and duration at 50% and 90% repolarization, maximum upstroke velocity, and effective refractory period, exhibited no significant alteration when cilazapril or cilazaprilate were administered at $10^{-8}-10^{-4}$ M.

These results indicate that in late arrhythmias without acute ischemia, ACE inhibitors may exert their preventive efficacy against sudden death not by direct effect on electrophysiological parameters but by indirect mechanisms, e.g., improvement in LV function, which is known to exert a decisive influence on mortality in patients with cardiac disease. In contrast, a number of antiarrhythmic drugs have been demonstrated to predominantly affect abnormal fibers rather than normal myocytes [7]. This selective action has yet to be incorporated into clinical practice, but may provide guidelines toward a more individual approach to antiarrhythmic drug therapy in cardiac failure.

Clinically, an association between the prevalence of spontaneous ventricular ectopy recorded by Holter monitoring and the risk of sudden death has been assumed by various studies, although this link is weakened by the high incidence of ventricular arrhythmias in most patients with impaired LV function [8–10]. This incidence appears to be related to a variety of contributing factors including:

1. Mechanical factors (regional wall motion stress)
2. Scarring
3. High catecholamines (increased sympathetic outflow/high levels of circulating catecholamines)
4. Electrolyte depletion
   K^+
   Mg^{++}
5. Drugs
   Diuretics
   Digitalis
   Phosphodiesterase inhibitors
   Antiarrhythmic drugs

No firm data have been presented so far to establish a correlation between a reduction in the incidence of ectopy brought about by antiarrhythmic drugs and an improvement in prognosis. The results of the above-mentioned CAST study rather suggest extremely cautious use of these drugs in asymptomatic patients with low-grade ventricular ectopy [11]. Although proarrhythmic action is the most feared mechanism of unwanted side effects of antiarrhythmic drugs [12, 13], the known negative inotropic action of antiarrhythmic agents may also prove fatal, particularly in patients with marginally compensated left-sided heart failure [14]. A schematic representation of this potentially vicious circle is presented in Fig. 3, while a comparison of the hemodynamic effects of antiarrhythmic drugs is shown in Table 1.

However, a significantly large group of patients is still considered to be at highest risk for sudden death, e.g., patients who have survived an aborted sudden death or emergency treatment for ventricular fibrillation or sustained ventricular tachycardia. In this high risk group, annual mortality ranges between 20% and 70%, resulting overwhelmingly from sudden cardiac death [15]. This poor prognosis has prompted the aggressive use of programmed electrical stimulation, designed to provoke the clinically documented arrhythmia by inducing ventricu-

Control

S₁ = 130 ms, VS = 30 ms S₂ = 130 ms CL = 132 ms 1s

ECG
LA eg
IZ epi 1
IZ epi 2
NZ epi 3
BP
20 mmHg

Cilazapril 1 mg/kg

S₁ = 130 ms, VS = 330 ms S₂ = 120 ms CL = 131 ms 1s

ECG
LA eg
IZ epi 1
IZ epi 2
NZ epi 3

Cilazapril 2 mg/kg

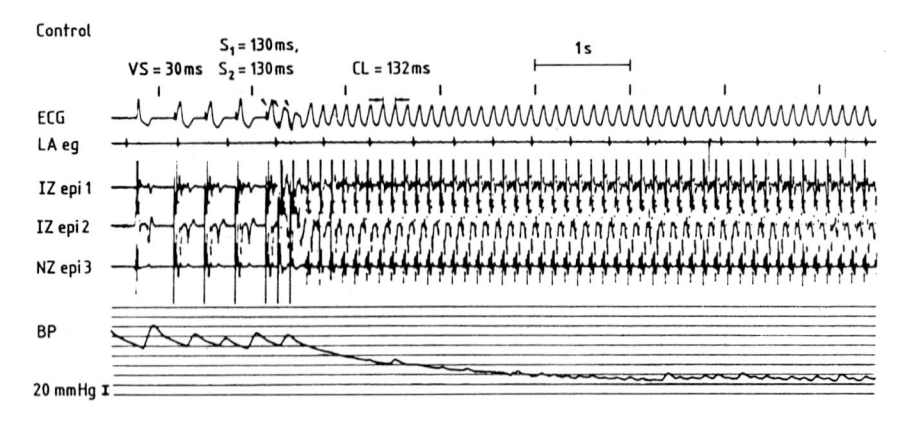

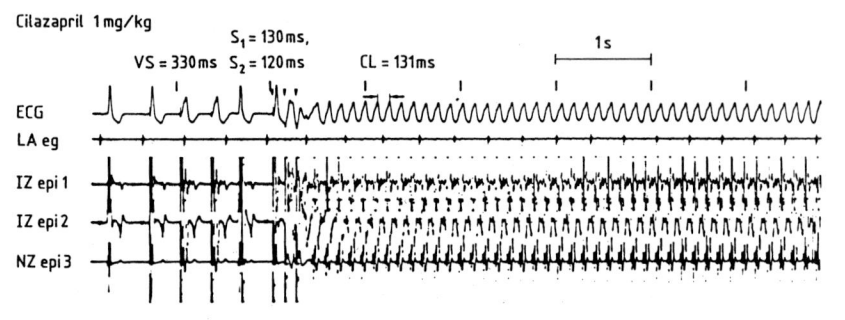

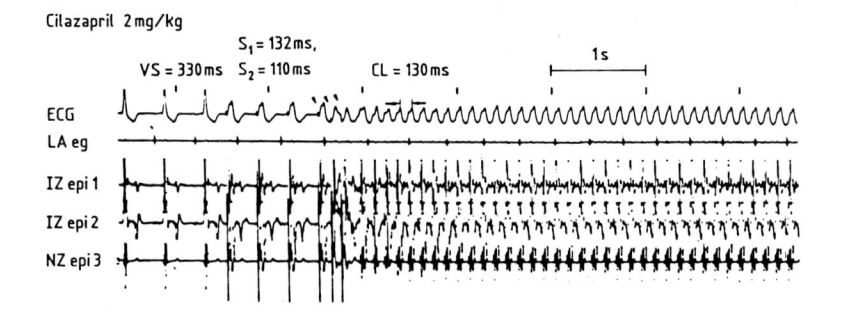

S₁ = 132 ms, VS = 330 ms S₂ = 110 ms CL = 130 ms 1s

ECG
LA eg
IZ epi 1
IZ epi 2
NZ epi 3

lar extrastimuli following a basic pacing train via temporary pacing catheters [16, 17].

The underlying concept is not only to investigate spontaneous ectopy which occurs more frequently but most likely only triggers the malignant event, but also to analyze electrical properties of the arrhythmia substrate, which is considered to provide suitable conditions for a sustained reentrant mechanism in most patients. The aim is to suppress patients' susceptibility to malignant arrhythmias by altering the electrical parameters of the assumed reentrant circuit and by directly investigating the influence of antiarrhythmic drugs. Because no drug has been shown to be effective in all patients, many electrophysiological centers prefer a

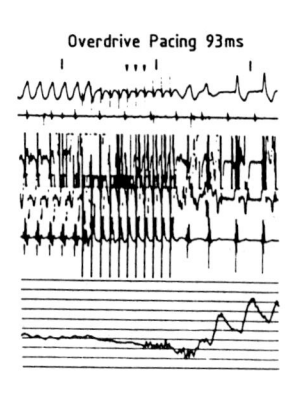

Fig. 2. Original tracing from an experiment with inducible monomorphic sustained ventricular tachycardia that could be reproducibly terminated by overdrive pacing. The middle and the low panels demonstrate the lack of efficacy of increasing doses of the ACE inhibitor cilazapril on both the rate of tachycardia and on termination of the tachycardia by overdrive pacing. Also, the morphology of the surface ECG and of intracardiac electrogram recordings remained unchanged

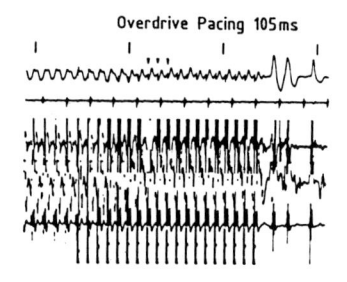

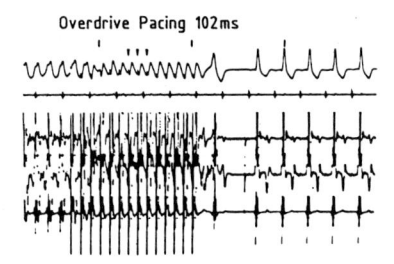

serial approach which allows comparative testing of various antiarrhythmic drugs within a relatively short period of time.

In order to test the efficacy of programmed electrical stimulation in patients with poor LV function, we studied 103 patients with dilative cardiomyopathy and malignant arrhythmias. All patients were investigated using a pacing protocol with basic driving cycles of 550 ms, 400 ms, and 330 ms employing a maximum of three extrastimuli. These patients were then subjected to serial drug testing consisting of the following antiarrhythmic drugs: quinidine (10 mg/kg, iv), propafenone (3 mg/kg, iv), mexiletine (5 mg/kg, iv), d-sotalol (1.5 mg/kg, iv), flecainide (2 mg/kg, iv), amiodarone (1 g/day for 10 days, orally). After either

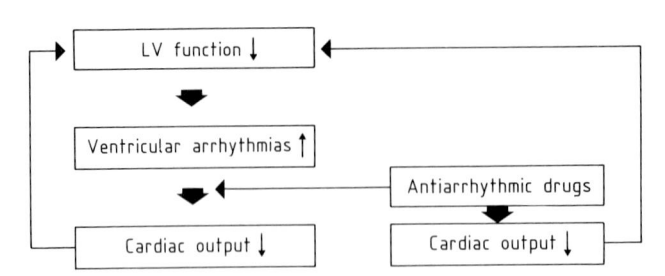

Fig. 3. Schematic diagram representing the possible beneficial and detrimental effects of antiarrhythmic drugs in patients with ventricular arrhythmias and heart failure

Table 1. Schematic representation of the hemodynamic effects of antiarrhythmic drugs on inotropy, peripheral resistance, and cardiac output[a]

			Inotropy	Peripheral resistance	Cardiac output
I	A	Quinidine	↓	↓↓	∅–(↓)
		Disopyramide	↓↓	↑	↓↓
		Procainamide	↓	↓	(↓)
	B	Lidocaine	(↓)	∅	∅
		Mexiletine	(↓)	∅	∅–(↓)
	C	Propafenone	↓	∅	(↓)
		Flecainide	↓	∅–↑	(↓)
II		β-receptor antagonists	↓↓	∅–↑	↓↓
III		Amiodarone	(↓)	↓	∅
		Sotalol	↓	∅	↓
		D-Sotalol	∅–(↓)	∅	∅
IV		Ca antagonists	↓	↓	∅–↓

[a] Antiarrhythmic drugs are listed according to the classification by Vaughan Williams. Note that most antiarrhythmic drugs present a more or less negative inotropic action while effects on peripheral resistance and cardiac output may differ quite considerably.

intravenous or oral treatment, the exact protocol of programmed stimulation at control was repeated. Only if no sustained arrhythmia, defined as lasting for at least 30 s or requiring termination because of hemodynamic side effects, was induced the drug was designated effective. Patients who remained inducible served as a control group. The overall success rate according to the electrophysiological criteria was 58% in the patients in whom long-term antiarrhythmic therapy had been initiated. The remaining patients received the antiarrhythmic agent that was causing the most prominent slowing of induced tachycardias, mostly amiodarone, which was administered in individual doses of 200–600 mg/day.

The clinical outcome in both groups, which did not differ significantly with respect to age (53 ± 12 vs 55 ± 17, responders vs nonresponders), ejection fraction ($31 \pm 12\%$ vs $27 \pm 16\%$), and clinical history, is demonstrated in Table 2. The responders did significantly better with a lower recurrence rate than the nonresponder group in which the recurrence rate was high. Similarly, the incidence of sudden death was lower in the responder group (4%/year) than in the nonrespon-

Table 2. Prognosis of patients with dilative cardiomyopathy obtained by serial drug testing

Group of patients	Prognosis	Rate (%/year)
Patients with suppression of inducibility by antiarrhythmic drugs	Low recurrence rate of arrhythmias	≈6
	Low incidence of sudden death	4
Patients without suppression of inducibility	High recurrence rate of arrhythmias	≈32
	High incidence of sudden death	18

der group (18%/year). This result, which is similar to the results of other studies of patients with coronary artery disease, can be interpreted in two ways. Firstly, the drugs may truly exert a beneficial action in preventing sudden death in the group of responders with their individual efficacy established by programmed stimulation, while the same group of drugs may simply fail or even exaggerate arrhythmias in the nonresponder group. Secondly, this response to arrhythmias may just provide a criterion for selecting patients with good and poor prognosis. This would imply that these patients could also do well when left without any antidysrhythmic therapy. However, no study has yet been presented to corroborate this assumption, though this might be a fascinating project. One has to keep in mind, however, that all patients in this group have already experienced one or more clinical episodes of malignant arrhythmias that were frequently aborted only by rather fortunate circumstances. Also, as mentioned before, most historical studies without antiarrhythmic drugs reported extremely high mortality. However, not only antiarrhythmic regimens have changed, but also medical therapy in general has been markedly improved most notably by the introduction of ACE inhibitors, which have already been unequivocally shown to reduce mortality.

Thus, the present use of antiarrhythmic drugs in patients with impaired cardiac function should be confined to patients with documented severe arrhythmias. It may be that programmed stimulation only serves to identify ineffective medication but it may also identify the group of patients who will benefit most either from cardiac transplant or implantable defibrillators with advanced antitachycardia function. These devices may lower the incidence of sudden death in the highest risk group, while avoiding major surgery and high expenses [18]. More research is required to finalize the role of drugs in this field for years to come.

References

1. Packer M (1985) Sudden unexpected death in patients with congestive heart failure: a second frontier. Circulation 72:681-685
2. Andeson KP, Freedman RA, Mason JW (1987) Sudden death in idiopathic cardiomyopathy. Ann Intern Med 107:104-106
3. Von Ohlshausen K, Schafer A, Mehmel HC, Schwarz F, Senges J, Kübler W (1984) Ventricular arrhythmias in idiopathic dilated cardiomyopathy. Br Heart J 51:195-201

4. The Cardiac Arrhythmia Suppression Trial (CAST) Investigators (1989) Preliminary report: effect of encainide and flecainide on mortality in a randomized trial of arrhythmia suppression after myocardial infarction. N Engl J Med 321:406–412
5. The CONSENSUS Trial Study Group (1987) Effects of enalapril on mortality in severe congestive heart failure. Results of the Cooperative North Scandinavian Enalapril Survival Study (CONSENSUS). N Engl J Med 316:1429–1435
6. Brachmann J, Kabell G, Scherlag BJ, Harrison L, Lazzara R (1983) Analysis of interectopic activation patterns during sustained ventricular tachycardia. Circulation 67:449–456
7. Lazzara R, El-Sherif N, Hope RR, Scherlag BJ (1978) Ventricular arrhythmias and electrophysiological consequences of myocardial ischemia and infarction. Circ Res 42:740–749
8. Dargie HJ, Cleland GF, Leckie BJ, Inglis CG, East BW, Ford I (1987) Relation of arrhythmias and electrolyte abnormalities to survival in patients with severe chronic heart failure. Circulation 75:IV-98–107
9. Meinertz T, Hofman T, Kasper W, Treese N, Bechtold H, Stienen U, Pop T, Leitner E-RV, Andresen D, Meyer J (1984) Significance of ventricular arrhythmias in dilated cardiomyopathy. Am J Cardiol 51:902–907
10. Wilson JR, Schwartz S, Sutton MS, Ferraro N, Horowitz LN, Reichek N, Josephson ME (1983) Prognosis in severe heart failure: Relation to hemodynamic measurements and ventricular ectopic activity. J Am Coll Cardiol 2:403–410
11. Francis GS (1988) Should asymptomatic ventricular arrhythmias in patients with congestive heart failure be treated with antiarrhythmic drugs? J Am Coll Cardiol 12:274–283
12. Brachmann J, Aidonidis I, Schöls W, Senges J, Kübler W (1986) Paradoxical arrhythmogenic properties of antiarrhythmic drugs – experimental and clinical finding. In: R Stroobandt, E Andries (eds) Cardiac arrhythmias. Elsevier, Amsterdam: 193–204
13. Minardo JD, Heger JJ, Miles WM, Zipes DP, Prystowsky EN (1988) Clinical characteristics of patients with ventricular fibrillation during antiarrhythmic therapy. N Engl J Med 319:257–262
14. Woosley RL (1987) Pharmacokinetics and pharmacodynamics of antiarrhythmic agents in patients with congestive heart failure. Am Heart J 114:1280–1291
15. Wilber DJ, Garan HS, Finkelstein D, Kelly E, Newell J, McGovern B, Ruskin JN (1988) Out-of-hospital cardiac arrest. Use of electrophysiologic testing in the prediction of long term outcome. N Engl J Med 318:19–24
16. Fisher JD, Cohen HL, Mehra R, et al. (1977) Cardiac pacing and pacemakers. II. Serial electrophysiologic-pharmacologic testing for control of recurrent tachyarrhythmias. Am Heart J 93:658–668
17. Josephson ME, Horowitz LN (1979) Electrophysiologic approach to therapy of recurrent sustained ventricular tachycardia. Am J Cardiol 43:631–642
18. Tchou PJ, Kadri N, Anderson J, Caceres JA, Jazayeri M, Akhtar M (1988) Automatic implantable cardioverter defibrillators and survival of patients with left ventricular dysfunction and malignant ventricular arrhythmias. Ann Intern Med 109:529–534

Nonpharmacologic Therapy for Malignant Ventricular Tachyarrhythmias in Patients with Congestive Heart Failure

S. Saksena

Malignant ventricular tachyarrhythmias constitute an important cause of sudden cardiac death in patients with congestive heart failure [25]. It is increasingly recognized that despite effective treatment of congestive heart failure, life-threatening ventricular tachyarrhythmias may abbreviate patient survial. The frequency of this complication impacts significantly on the overall clinical outcome of these patients. In some instances, the therapeutic agent chosen for the treatment of congestive heart failure, for example, certain inotropic agents, may actually aggravate the ventricular tachyarrhythmia [23]. Surgical therapy in patients with congestive heart failure is also not immune to this complication. It is well-established that patients who have undergone aortic valve replacement for severe aortic valvular stenosis may experience postoperative sudden cardiac death. Clinical studies have suggested an association with the presence of complex ventricular tachyarrhythmias and nonsustained ventricular tachycardia (VT) on Holter monitoring. Similarly, patients who have undergone visually guided resection of a ventricular aneurysm or non-map-guided surgical resection of ventricular myocardium have a higher risk of recurrent postoperative ventricular tachyarrhythmias than patients who have undergone map-directed operations [40]. Finally, the presence of complex ventricular tachyarrhythmias or nonsustained VT in patients with left ventricular dysfunction due to a variety of anatomic abnormalities is an independent predictor of sudden cardiac death. While the majority of information available is in patients with coronary artery disease, increasing information is now available in patients with dilated cardiomyopathy, hypertrophic cardiomyopathy, and certain types of valvular heart disease [15].

Approaches to antiarrhythmic treatment in this patient population have included the use of empiric antiarrhythmic drug therapy or directed antiarrhythmic drug therapy alone or combined with non-pharmacological approaches. Empiric antiarrhythmic drug therapy has not been shown to reduce the incidence of sudden cardiac death in patients treated with this approach in a variety of anatomic substrates. Recent data from The Cardiac Arrhythmia Suppression Trial suggest that empiric therapy with certain group Ic antiarrhythmic agents may actually increase the incidence of sudden cardiac arrest or recurrent ventricular tachyarrhythmias [8]. The proarrhythmic potential of these particular agents is particularly prominent in patients with advanced left ventricular dysfunction. Directed antiarrhythmic therapy can be planned on the basis of noninvasive approaches such as ambulatory electrocardiographic monitoring or invasive approaches such as electrophysiological evaluation. While suppression of ventricular ectopic activity can be quantitated by the ambulatory electrocardiographic approach, simple suppression of ectopic activity quantitatively may not predict a favorable outcome. However, suppression of complex ventricular ectopic activity and nonsustained VT can provide a more favorable prognosis using this approach. This has been validated with certain antiarrhythmic agents such as amiodarone in patients with left ventricular dysfunction [20, 48]. However, the extent of arrhythmia control is achieved on the basis of ambulatory electrocardiographic monitoring, and patient survival is usually inferior to that obtained by directed invasive approaches such as electrophysiological evaluation [20]. Particularly relevant is the fact that a large number of patients with sustained ventricular tachyarrhythmias fail to manifest significant ventricular ectopic activity on ambulatory electrocardiographic monitoring. In a recent multicenter trial sponsored by the National Institutes of Health, only 27% of patients with sustained VT or ventricular fibrillation were candidates for both noninvasive and invasive approaches [12]. These data would suggest that a larger proportion of patients are candidates for the invasive approach, but neither approach can be used exclusively in all patients. Directed antiarrhythmic therapy on the basis of electrophysiological evaluation has been shown to have a favorable outcome during long-term follow-up in patients with sustained VT, ventricular fibrillation, and/or cardiac arrest [50]. Follow-up of patients who failed to achieve control of the ventricular tachyarrhythmia based on electrophysiological evaluation shows that the clinical outcome of this group of patients is poor, with a high incidence of recurrent cardiac arrest [50]. In identifying the factors that select patients who do not achieve control with directed antiarrhythmic therapy, advanced left ventricular dysfunction is a primary determinant. Finally, the incidence of proarrhythmic effects of antiarrhythmic agents, particularly type Ic agents, are highest in the population with sustained VT and left ventricular dysfunction [10]. Thus, it can be appreciated that the likelihood of identifying successful antiarrhythmic drug therapy in a patient population with heart failure and sustained VT or ventricular fibrillation is reduced. Complicating the clinical dilemma is a well-established clinical observation that sustained ventricular tachyarrhythmias are most frequently observed in patients with myocardial disease and ventricular dysfunction. The need for alternative forms of antiarrhythmic therapy, i.e., nonpharmacologic approaches, becomes self-evident from this constellation of observations.

Nonpharmacologic approaches to antiarrhythmic therapy employ two general strategies, namely, elimination of the arrhythmogenic substrate (ablation) or immediate reversion of sustained ventricular tachyarrhythmias by implantable electronic devices such as cardioverter-defibrillators. Ablation of the arrhythmogenic substrate can be accomplished by catheter-delivered destructive energy or by surgical removal or destruction of involved tissues intraoperatively. Energy sources employed for catheter ablation studies have included passive contact and active fixation catheter delivery systems [1]. Different combinations of ablative energy and delivery systems have been evaluated in a variety of different anatomic substrates. Intraoperative techniques for ablation of VT substrates have ranged from simple incision or excision of infarcted tissue, subendocardial resection, exclusion of involved tissues by encircling endocardial ventriculotomy, or physical ablation of the substrate using cryothermal or laser techniques [4, 7, 29, 36]. Reversion of sustained ventricular tachyarrhythmia by implantable electronic devices has been achieved by pacing techniques and delivery of epicardial or endocardial shocks [14, 24, 31, 51]. A variety of pulse generators able to deliver pacing therapy, low-energy and high-energy shocks have been used in conjunction with epicardial and endocardial electrode systems. Each of these approaches is in various stages of development and/or clinical evaluation. A few have achieved the stature of routine clinical practice.

Ablation of the arrhythmogenic substrate has initially attempted using an empiric surgical approach. This approach has been largely abandoned due to the uncertain results with respect to arrhythmia control. This has been largely related to failure of accurate intraoperative identification of the arrhythmogenic substrate. Experimental and clinical studies utilizing cardiac mapping techniques have suggested that the sites of origin of ventricular tachyarrhythmias may lie in the transitional zone of a myocardial infarction at the margins of ventricular aneurysm or infarct [18]. Reentry is believed to originate in surviving cells which are scattered and interspersed with fibrotic regions in these tissues. In patients with noncoronary disease, there is less characterization of the anatomic substrate. Intraoperative mapping studies confirm the presence of slowly conducting diseased tissues in these regions. Diastolic electrical activity during sustained VT has been demonstrated both in subendocardial layers and endocardium but also in epicardial recordings [19, 30]. Early studies demonstrated disparity in the site of earliest ventricular activation as detected by endocardial and epicardial recordings. However, in more recent studies, our experience has shown the presence of epicardial diastolic electrical activities often parallels endocardial diastolic electrical activity in the left ventricular free wall regions. Tachycardias arising in the septal region, however, show marked discordance between epicardial and endocardial recordings are usually used to guide ablation. Finally, recent studies using plunge electrodes suggest the presence of intramural sites of reentry in a significant number of patients [5]. Thus, any ablative technique that is exceptionally focal in its effects may either fail to interrupt the tachycardia circuit or leave alternative pathways behind for continuation of the same or other tachycardias. Frequently, these anatomic paths may be in close proximity to the ablated site. Experience with laser ablation of VT intraoperatively suggest that an average of 9 cm^2 of endocardial and subendocardial tissues with a depth of 3–4 mm may be necessary for successful elimination of sufficient arrhythmogenic substrate for a single VT morphology [41]. It is, however, our experience that considerable variability can be encountered in the size of the substrate for individual tachycardias. The coexistence of multiple potential tachycardia circuits in a single patient further confounds the issue. Ablation of multiple morphologies of tachycardia is usually necessary for satisfactory results [41].

Map-directed approaches for ablation of the arrhythmogenic substrate have provided superior results to non-map-directed approaches. Complexity of preoperative and intraoperative cardiac mapping techniques associated with absence of appropriate user-friendly instrumentation has greatly retarded the development of intraoperative map-guided surgery. Early attempts using single epicardial and endocardial recordings during induced ventricular tachycardia were tedious and time consuming and have now been replaced by the use of multiple simultaneous electrogram recordings during the tachyarrhythmia. This is achieved by use of multiple electrode arrays such as plaque electrodes, epicardial sock electrodes, plunge electrodes, endocardial balloon electrodes, and ribbon electrodes. This has greatly expedited data acquisition. Data analysis, however, remains a tedious, physician-observer dependent task. More recently, computerized acquisition and analytic techniques are being applied to this effort [11]. Since intraoperative ventricular mapping is usually performed on partial or full cardiopulmonary bypass, it is generally desirable to perform this expeditiously. In our experience, we attempt to limit actual cardiac mapping time to 30 min or less. However, the time required for induction of VT during general anesthesia and after cardiac manipulation often prolongs this effort.

Ablative techniques that are in current use range from subendocardial resection, encircling endocardial ventriculotomy, or extended endocardial resection to physical ablation techniques such as cryothermal ablation and laser ablation. Combination approaches have been used. Extensive experience is now available with several of these approaches and has been well summarized in a recent international registry [4]. Subendocardial resection has been reported to be associated with long-term arrhythmia control in approximately 75%–80% of patients. Approximately two-thirds of these patients during follow-up have been free of postoperative antiarrhythmic drug therapy whereas approximately one-third continue to require antiarrhythmic drugs. Perioperative mortality for this procedure has ranged from 8% to 15% [4, 22, 34]. In most of these series, subendocardial resection has been performed in conjunction with coronary artery bypass surgery and/or ventricular aneurysmectomy. In our experience, the success rate of subendocardial resection has been similar to those at other centers. Perioperative mortality was 8%. On long-term follow-up, one-third of patients still required postoperative antiarrhythmic drug therapy. In analyzing the results it became apparent that patients with inferior, posterior, and septal sites of origin of VT had higher failure rates as judged by electrophysiologic testing postoperatively than patients with anterior or lateral sites of origin. Modifications are being introduced in an attempt to improve these results. These included encirclement of the base of the papillary muscle by the surgical incision in that region, or cryothermal ablation. Alternative operations such as encircling endocardial ventriculotomy, which may not be map-directed, have had significant success rates in arrhythmia suppression but have been associated with significant myocardial dysfunction postoperatively, often related to the need for extensive ablation in patients with severely compromised left ventricular function [4]. Cryothermal ablation has also been associated with good arrhythmia control, but data from the international registry suggested poor survival, perhaps again related to the extensive myocardial ablation [4]. Furthermore, cryothermal techniques are slow and time consuming. Exclusive cryothermal ablation of VT sites may take 30 min or more in patients with multiple tachycardia sites. Since perioperative risk is related to several factors including intraoperative events such as the length of cardiopulmonary bypass, abbreviation of the ablation procedure is as desirable as a brief mapping procedure. Finally, recent data suggest that surgical approaches in patients with noncoronary disease may be applicable to a limited number of patients. While they are frequently applied to arrhythmogenic right ventricular dysplasia, longer experience has initiated discussions of the merits of medical and surgical therapy. Patients with diffuse cardiomyopathic processes including dilated cardiomyopathy or hypertrophic cardiomyopathy may not provide the focal substrate essential to a surgical ablative procedure. The role of surgical ablation in these disease substrates remains to be established.

In an effort to overcome the limitations of current surgical procedures, we undertook a developmental program for the use of laser energy for intraoperative ablation of ventricular and supraventricular tachyarrhythmias. Experimental studies demonstrated the feasibility of controlled myocardial ablation with pulsed argon laser energy [8]. Furthermore, ablation of normal and diseased human ventricular myocardium was feasible with this technique [33]. Quantitative relationships between the extent of ablation and amount of delivered energy could be established in normal ventricular myocardium within defined limits and, to a lesser extent, in diseased ventricular myocardium. We undertook clinical evaluation of this technique approximately 4 years ago. Intraoperative mapping was performed using multipolar plaque electrodes for epicardial and endocardial mapping during induced VT [36]. The arrhythmogenic substrate was identified by the presence of mid-diastolic and presystolic electrical activity during the induced arrhythmia [36]. Intraoperative ablation was attempted with transcatheter pulsed argon laser discharges delivered to the ventricular endocardium through an air medium. A series of pulsed laser lesions were performed in a congruent fashion to achieve a confluent endocardial ablated zone (Fig. 1). While laser ablation was performed in a normothermic beating heart, it was attempted during induced VT [41]. Termination of incessant sustained VT was demonstrated in a few patients

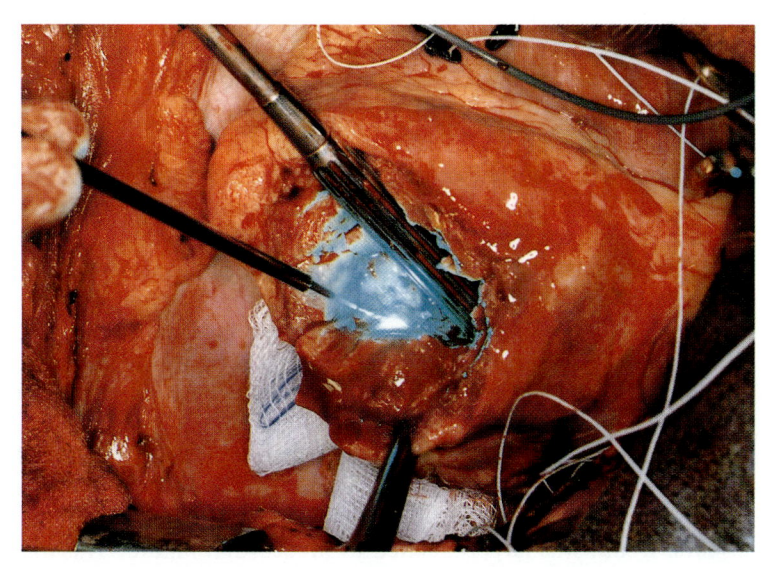

Fig. 1. Endocardial ablation of ventricular tachycardia substrate in a patient with coronary artery disease. Preoperative and intraoperative mapping localized the site of ventricular tachycardia origin to the posterior wall of the left ventricule in this patient. Intraoperative pulsed argon laser radiation to the left ventricular endocardium at this site was used for endocardial ablation. Note the transcatheter delivery of laser energy that produces a series of adjoining endocardial lesions

in vivo. In most instances, however, laser ablation was performed in a normothermic heart during sinus rhythm after mapping had been performed during the induced tachycardia. This was largely related to the inability to maintain sustained VT through the surgical procedure. Initial reports demonstrated feasibility and safety of the technique [29, 36]. Long-term experience is now available and reported with this approach [41]. The initial 20 patients had coronary artery disease with a mean left ventricular ejection fraction of 34% and mean cardiac index of $2.9 \, l \, min^{-1} \, m^{-2}$. Sites of VT origin were obtained from preoperative and intraoperative mapping. A mean of 1.9 VT morphologies were mapped per patient. The majority of the VT sites were located in the septum, inferior, and posterior wall, consistent with data obtained from the international registry. The majority of VT morphologies (80%) were ablated with laser energy alone and the remainder with laser ablation combined with mechanical endocardial resection. The mean area of laser ablation was $9 \pm 6 \, cm^2$, and the mean energy density was $313 \pm 125 \, J/cm^2$. A majority of the patients (80%) underwent concomitant coronary artery bypass surgery. Perioperative mortality in the initial series was 5%. There was no sudden death in the initial 12 months of complete follow-up. One patient (5%) who was lost to follow-up reportedly died of myocardial infarction. One patient died of unrelated medical disease in the 2nd month of follow-up. Total survival was 85% with a mean follow-up duration of 14 ± 8 months. Of the surviving patients, 95% require no antiarrhythmic drug therapy. This is a significant improvement from prior reports. Efficacy rates for inferior, septal, and posterior sites of VT origin have been markedly improved by laser ablation (95%) as compared to subendocardial resection (55%) in our experience. Since the largest proportion of patients have these sites of VT origin, this approach could widened the patient population and range of tachyarrhythmias suitable for surgical ablation. Factors predicting the failure of the subendocardial resection technique have been identified. Inferior and posterior left ventricular sites of VT origin, multiple induced VT morphologies, disparate sites of VT origin, absence of a discrete left ventricular aneurysm, and right bundle branch block VT morphology have been associated with failure. Initial experience with laser ablation suggests that these predictors of failure with subendocardial resection can be addressed by this technique. Another advantage of the laser technique is the effect of the laser energy on the target arrhythmia can be judged intraoperatively in some patients. Failure to achieve arrhythmia elimination during normothermic irradiation of target tissues can permit alteration of the surgical procedure and result in the need for continued mapping or ablation. This is not possible with mechanical techniques. Thus, the laser technique can be used to define intraoperatively the extent of its anatomic and electrophysiologic effects. This is not often possible with other techniques. The long-term survival of cryothermal procedures for VT ablation in one large multicenter report was 62% at 1 year and 55% at 2 years. Death was largely related to myocardial failure. This may be related to the fact that cryosurgery does not eliminate disease tissues but converts normal tissue to dense scar which may account for the left ventricular dysfunction.

The current role of intraoperative ablation techniques in patients with ventricular tachyarrhythmias and congestive heart failure can now be defined based upon our and other reported experiences. This technique is most applicable to patients with coronary artery disease with left ventricular ejection fractions ranging from 20% to 40%. Results in patients with global left ventricular ejection fractions below 20% are disappointing. While the arrhythmia may be successfully suppressed postoperatively, long-term survival is limited. The presence of a focal anatomic abnormality such as ventricular aneurysm or myocardial infarction makes the patient particularly suitable for this approach. However, we have observed well-defined infarction zones intraoperatively in patients whose preoperative left ventricular angiograms did not demonstrate such clearly defined anatomic abnormalities. Presence of a ventricular tachyarrhythmia that is suitable for cardiac mapping is essential to such an approach. Preoperative risk factors in our experience include the presence of diabetes mellitus and renal failure. Preoperative evaluation of renal and hematologic status is recommended. We have avoided these procedures in patients over 75 years of age. While these limitations do not preclude surgical ablation, they provide general guidelines for patient selection. Careful and complete cardiac mapping of all induced ventricular tachycardia morphologies is recommended. Presence of obstructive coronary artery disease amenable to bypass surgery can further improve survival in this group of patients with advanced coronary disease and poor left ventricular function [8]. Finally, correction of anatomic abnormalities by procedures such as a ventricular aneurysmectomy may also resolve symptoms and signs of congestive heart failure and improve the functional status of the patient. Such an approach thus permits surgical therapy of both the primary disease with its manifestation of congestive heart failure and life-threatening ventricular arrhythmias. Contraindications to this approach, in my view, include patients with diffuse myocardial disease, multiple and pleomorphic ventricular tachycardias, inability to map VT preoperatively or intraoperatively, and patients with advanced systemic diseases including renal and pulmonary disease.

In the past decade, alternative approaches to intraoperative ablation of the arrhythmogenic substrate have been examined. Transcatheter delivery of ablative energy to achieve a similar outcome has been developed [16, 44]. This approach has many of the same considerations as have been discussed above for surgical ablation. Careful mapping and identification of the arrhythmogenic substrate remains a key issue. This becomes a greater challenge due to the absence of visual guidance during this procedure. Cardiac catheterization techniques with fluoroscopic imaging are used instead. Electrode catheters are directed to the arrhythmogenic substrate which is electrically identified. In some instances, cine angiography is used to confirm electrode position. Subsequently, ablative energy is delivered preferably via specially designed catheters at that site. This approach has been most successfully used for ablation of the specialized conduction system located at the right atrioventricular junction in order to control supraventricular tachyarrhythmias. In a recent report of a multicenter registry, transcatheter direct current shock ablation was used to interrupt or modify atrioventricular conduction in patients with supraventricular tachycardia [13]. Successful interruption of atrioventricular conduction was achieved in 64% who subsequently required cardiac pacing. Modification of atrioventricular conduction resulting in control of tachycardia rate without the use of antiarrhythmic drugs could be achieved in a further 9% of patients whereas control with previously ineffective antiarrhythmic drugs could be achieved in an additional 12% of patients. The procedure can be used on more than one occasion if it is unsuccessful on the first attempt. The procedure-related complications were 0.5%. The procedure itself requires transient general anesthesia during direct current shock application and temporary pacing followed by permanent pacing thereafter. Catheter direct current shock ablation has also been applied to other arrhythmogenic substrates such as accessory atrioventricular bypass tracts and ventricular tachycardia foci. Significant concerns arose when direct current shocks were applied for ablation of left-sided accessory pathways via the coronary sinus. Coronary sinus rupture with hemopericardium and cardiac tamponade have been reported. In an effort to overcome these limitations, alternative approaches such as endocardial shock delivery using either transeptal or retrograde catheterization techniques permitting delivery of direct current shocks at the left atrioventricular junction have been used [49]. In addition, these techniques are now being increasingly used for ablation along the tricuspid annulus. The complication rate related to the procedure as well as the long-term efficacy and safety of these techniques remains to be defined. In patients with refractory ventricular tachycardia, multiple high-energy direct current shocks have been delivered through this transcatheter technique to the arrhythmogenic substrate. The arrhythmogenic substrate has been identified by the catheter endocardial mapping techniques. It is now suggested that sites of mid-diastolic and presystolic activity forming the slowly conducting pathway in the reentrant circuit should be the target tissue. Multiple high-energy shocks are usually required for successful ablation. However, the success rate for ablation reported from the international registry data is considerably lower than that described for supraventricular tachycardia [13]. Less than one-fourth of patients have successful suppression of their ventricular tachyarrhythmia without the need for postoperative antiarrhythmic drug therapy. Another third may be responsive to previously ineffective drugs, but the long-term results in this group remain unknown. Finally, up to 40% of patients and perhaps more are uncontrolled with this approach. The procedure-related complications are considerably higher and have been as high as 20% in some reports. A procedure-related mortality rate of approximately 5% has been suggested. In view of these results, mapping-guided surgical ablation techniques offer much higher cure rates with only a slightly higher procedure-related mortality. They are therefore recommended as the first line of treatment for patients with VT who are appropriate candidates for this techniques.

It has been recognized that the limited efficacy of catheter direct current shock ablation in patients with VT may be related to the inability of direct current shocks to effectively ablate in diseased, particularly fibrotic, ventricular myocardium. In addition, the immediate procedure-related complications may be related to the barotraumatic effects of such shocks. When delivered in thin-walled cardiac structures such as the coronary sinus or atrium, perforation may occur due to this property. In order to overcome these limitations of direct current shocks alternative ablative energy sources are being examined. High-frequency current which can produce myocardial ablation by thermal effects and current delivery has been proposed [1, 17]. This technique has no barotraumatic effects and can be applied in awake, unanesthetized patients. While formal data in a substantial number of patients are unavailable, early reports suggest that this technique may be valuable for right atrioventricular junctional ablation, and efficacy rates using pooled data appear to approach 50% [46]. Further innovations in catheter delivery systems, modes of energy delivery and mapping could enhance efficacy. However, high-frequency current has very limited effects in diseased/fibrotic ventricular myocardium and has been largely inefficacious in VT ablation from early data [1, 46]. Improvements in catheter delivery systems have been considered for both high-frequency energy delivery and direct current shock delivery. While the majority of ablation techniques have used passive contact ring electrodes mounted in the center of cardiac catheters, more recently specialized catheter delivery systems have been developed. A suction electrode catheter that can attach itself to the target tissue has been examined [39]. In experimental studies, we have observed successful ablation of the right atrioventricular junction in canine experiments with low-eneregy direct current shocks which have few barotraumatic effects. In addition, delivery of high-frequency current through these suction electrodes has been attempted, and successful experimental and clinical ablation has been achieved in occasional instances [1]. Large surface area electrode catheters have been proposed for high-frequency ablation, thermistor-tipped temperature-controlled energy systems are under development [3]. Another alternative energy source being evaluated is laser energy. From the intraoperative ablation experience, laser energy has been shown to successfully ablate normal as well as diseased ventricular myocardium. Transcatheter delivery using fiberoptics during intraoperative procedures has been successfully demonstrated [26]. Experimental studies have now looked at transcatheter ablation of the atrioventricular junction and ventricular myocardium using laser energy. While laser energy produces a large amount of its effects because of thermal effects, selective absorption techniques can also be considered.

In patients with refractory congestive heart failure, catheter ablation techniques are most commonly applied to patients with atrial fibrillation or VT. Supraventricular tachyarrhythmias causing decompensation of congestive heart failure are frequent, and control of ventricular rate using antiarrhythmic drug therapy is often difficult. Resolution of congestive heart failure may aid control of ventricular rate, particularly in patients with refractory atrial fibrillation. However, resolution of congestive heart failure may not be feasible in the presence of atrial fibrillation with rapid ventricular rates. Thus, in refractory patients, atrioventricular junctional ablation using catheter techniques is frequently applied. Control of ventricular rate is achieved, and either a rate responsive ventricular demand pacemaker, or in patients with intact sinus mechanisms, atrioventricular sequential pacing may be utilized. This may assist in better control of congestive heart failure. Similarly, the initial presentation of sustained VT or ventricular fibrillation may occur during a period of exacerbation of congestive heart failure. Alternatively, increased frequency of such episodes may be observed during worsening congestive heart failure or after intensive diuretic therapy for heart failure resulting in hypokalemia and hypomagnesemia. Treatment of the ventricular tachyarrhythmia includes resolution of the heart failure, correction of electrolyte and acid-base abnormalities as well as directed antiarrhythmic therapy. Catheter ablation of incessant VT may assist in management in selected patients.

The alternative nonpharmacologic approach to antiarrhythmic therapy in sustained VT or ventricular fibrillation involves reversion of the manifest arrhythmia. This is usually achieved by delivery of electrical therapy after arrhythmia detection. While sustained VT may or may not be associated with hemodynamic collapse or symptoms, sustained ventricular fibrillation results in cardiocirculatory collapse within a few seconds of its onset. Thus, while selected patients with VT may be aware of their arrhythmia without severe cardiocirculatory disturbances and could manually trigger electrical therapy, the vast majority of patients need automated arrhythmia detection and termination. Thus, while early reports exist of patient-activated pacing or low-energy shock cardioversion of VT, application of this approach to the general patient population with VT or ventricular fibrillation only became possible with the development of an implantable cardioverter-defibrillator with automated detection and therapy delivery [14, 24, 51]. The implantable pulse generator continuously monitors heart rate and electrogram morphology. When detection criteria are met, the device delivers a high energy (30–35 J) direct current shock [24]. Electrogram acquisition and shock delivery is currently achieved by using a pair of epicardial screw-in electrodes for the former purpose and epicardial patch electrodes for the latter purpose. This results in the need for a thoracotomy for lead placement. Optimal sensing lead placement is determined by analyzing electrogram amplitude and morphology during induced VT or ventricular fibrillation at intraoperative electrophysiologic testing. Optimal patch electrode placement is determined by seeking the lowest reliable defibrillation threshold during induced ventricular fibrillation. Defibrillation thresholds are measured using an external cardioverter-defibrillator and values below 15–20 J are customary. The defibrillation leads are placed intrapericardially or extrapericardially and are tunneled to an abdominal pocket where the pulse generator is implanted. A variety of surgical approaches including a median sternotomy, lateral thoracotomy, subxiphoid or subcostal incisions have been employed. The perioperative morbidity and mortality of this technique in patients with sustained ventricular tachyarrhythmias and advanced cardiac disease is significant. Some centers have reported mortality as low as 2% or 3%; other centers, depending on their patient population, have had rates of 6%–8%. Our 6-year experience in a patient population with significant left ventricular dysfunction and heart failure has been 7%. The long-term arrhythmic or sudden death rate has been below 5%. This has largely been related to system failures in a few patients. Similar data from other centers as well as pooled international data suggest that the arrhythmic death rate is below 3% annually [45]. This has a significant impact on the total mortality in patients with severe organic heart disease and sustained VT or ventricular fibrillation. This improvement in arrhythmic death rates, however, does not obviate other causes of cardiac and noncardiac deaths in this population. Total, while reduced, 80% at 3 years and 70% at 5 years. The major cause of mortality in this patient population is refractory congestive heart failure in our experience. Thus, aggressive treatment of congestive heart failure remains the second major therapeutic intervention necessary to enhance patient survival.

Several limitations in the currently approved device and lead systems are apparent from clinical experience. In addition to the perioperative risk of implantation, long-term patient tolerance of high-energy shock therapy for cardioversion and defibrillation has been limited. Limited longevity of currently implantable pulse generators (2–3 years) as well as nonprogrammability, limitations in arrhythmia detection algorithms, and pulse generator size and cost have contributed to a slow acceptance of this therapeutic approach [28]. Recent improvements are designed to address these issues [37]. While a catheter-based defibrillation lead system was contemplated over a decade ago, reliable catheter defibrillation and cardioversion was not achieved in early attempts. Over the past several years, we evaluated the factors determining the outcome of catheter cardioversion and defibrillation as well as the mechanisms of successful and unsuccessful conversion [9, 38]. Dual endocardial electrode systems using right ventricular and right atrial defibrillation electrodes were unable to reliably convert rapid VT or ventricular fibrillation [27]. Furthermore, energies of 10 J or less were quite ineffective in this regard [6]. A prospective randomized controlled study showed that low-energy cardioversion shocks were rarely more effective than rapid ventricular pacing, and that efficacy of endocardial cardioversion increased with increasing energy [9, 32]. Successful conversion was dependent on penetration and depolarization of critical diastolic elements in the tachycardia circuit. This could be achieved by increasing shock energy or energy distribution. The former approach is feasible up to the limitations imposed by the size and output of the current implantable pulse generator.

Thus, we examined alternative electrode configurations for improved spatial distribution of shock energy. Inclusion of the left ventricle was deemed important in this approach. In 1985, we evaluated a bidirectional shock technique using a triple-electrode system in humans [21, 35]. A right ventricular common cathode was used with dual anodes placed in the right atrium and the left thorax. In early clinical testing, a left thoracic skin patch electrode was used in a variety of locations including left infraclavicular, left lateral, left posterior and at the cardiac apex. A single shock was delivered using this triple-electrode system and established dual current pathways (Fig. 2). Energy transmission from the right ventric-

Fig. 2. Bidirectional shock delivered using a triple-electrode system for endocardial cardioversion and defibrillation. Two catheter electrodes are introduced into the right heart. These can be a single or separate catheters. A right ventricular common cathode was used. A right atrial anode as well as a left thoracic patch electrode are cross-connected and used as dual anodes. A single shock is then delivered which establishes dual current pathways (*interrupted lines*)

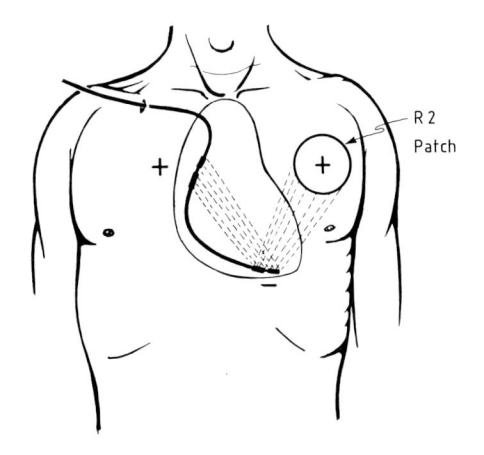

ular–right atrial electrodes as well as right ventricular–left thoracic patch electrodes was demonstrated [35]. Catheter electrode size was also important in energy distribution. Small surface area catheter electrodes could successfully be used for cardioversion of rapid VT using bidirectional shocks [21]. However, reproducible defibrillation could not be demonstrated. A large surface area right ventricular cathode and right atrial anode was then used in conjunction with the left thoracic patch electrode, and preliminary studies demonstrated the feasibility of defibrillation of this approach. We undertook implantation of this triple-electrode system of endocardial defibrillation in 1987 [31]. The first implant reported in January 1988 demonstrated the feasibility of this approach. Successful out-of-hospital conversion of rapid VT was demonstrated in this patient. Subsequently, a multicenter clinical trial was initiated. The early clinical experience continued to demonstrate reliable endocardial defibrillation with this triple-electrode technique. A variety of endocardial defibrillation electrode configurations using dual- and triple-electrode systems was also tested in this trial. The highest yield for successful endocardial defibrillation was obtained with a triple-electrode system using a right ventricular cathode and dual anodes in the right atrium and left thorax, as noted in our previous work. In our initial clinical series, we reported a mean endocardial defibrillation threshold of 18 J with this lead system [43]. In nine out of ten patients in whom an endocardial defibrillation lead system implant was attempted this was successfully performed. This yield was somewhat higher than in the multicenter study (69%) [2].

Considerable attention was paid in our implant to define the optimal patch electrode position with an external skin patch electrode being used to define the subcutaneous patch electrode location. Figure 3 is the schematic diagram of the implant technique. While a single catheter electrode was used with two defibrillation electrodes in this study, subsequent developments have led to the trial of a variety of different right ventricular defibrillation cathode configurations as well as the use of smaller flexible pacing defibrillation leads. Early clinical experience demonstrated the feasibility of endocardial defibrillation on a chronic basis. Successful out-of-hospital conversion of sustained VT and ventricular fibrillation has been demonstrated. However, lead conductor fracture in the lead body resulted in system failures and one reported sudden death. Alternative approaches using separate leads for right ventricular cathode and right atrial anode are being considered [42]. Modification of current dual chamber pacing lead systems to permit bipolar endocardial pacing, sensing, and defibrilaltion are being evaluated. The perioperative risk of implantation was markedly reduced. In our experience, the majority of patients had had prior cardiac surgery or had advanced systemic diseases that would make a thoracotomy particularly hazardous. There was no implant mortality and minimal morbidity. The multicenter experience also did not demonstrate significant perioperative mortality. It can be reasonably expected that chronic use of endocardial defibrillation lead systems will markedly reduce the perioperative risk associated with implantation of a cardioverter-defibrillator. The long-term clinical efficacy and safety of this approach is currently under evaluation.

The other major limitations of cardioverter-defibrillator therapy related to the pulse generator are similarly being addressed. A new generation of multipro-

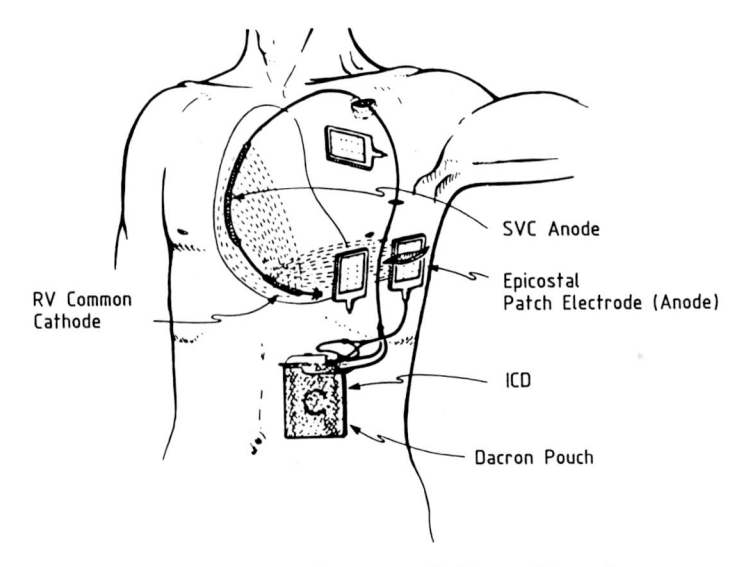

Fig. 3. Schematic diagram of implantation of a cardioverter-defibrillator without thoracotomy using a triple-electrode system. A single tripolar catheter with two defibrillation electrodes and one tip-sensing electrode is advanced from the left subclavian vein to the right ventricular apex. A left thoracic patch is placed submuscularly at different possible site on the left thorax as shown. The right ventricular electrode is used as a common cathode, and dual anodes in the superior vena cava and right atrium and the patch electrode are cross-connected by a Y-connector. The implantable defibrillator is placed in an abdominal pouch. *RV*, Right ventricular; *SVC*, superior vena cava; *AICD*, implantable cardioverter-defibrillator. (Modified from [1] with permission from JAMA)

grammable devices with pacing and shock therapy as well as programmable arrhythmia detection algorithms is currently under study. We have implanted two such systems, the Telectronics Guardian Series Models 4201 and 4202 (Telectronics Pacing Systems, Denver, CO) and the Ventak P (Cardiac Pacemakers, Minneapolis, MN) programmable pulse generators. The former permits pacing, cardioversion, and defibrillation whereas the latter has capabilities for cardioversion and defibrillation programmability alone. Sensing is programmable to a limited extent. Currently used with epicardial lead systems, both devices are capable of being interfaced with endocardial lead systems in the future. Initial clinical experience suggests that programmability can be frequently used during follow-up to reduce system complications. Figure 4 is an example of using individualized therapies for cardioversion and defibrillation. In this patient, sustained VT could be terminated with a 3-J shock (panel a) whereas ventricular fibrillation could be terminated with a 13-J shock (panel b). The Telectronics Guardian Model 4202 can deliver a train of seven shocks, of which the initial shock is programmable. Depending on the clinical manifestation of the patient being VT or ventricular fibrillation, the initial shock energy can be set. In the initial three implants, out-of-hospital VT conversion has been demonstrated in two patients, and successful resuscitation from out-of-hospital cardiac arrest has occurred in the third patient. Efforts to reduce defibrillation thresholds continue for endocardial lead

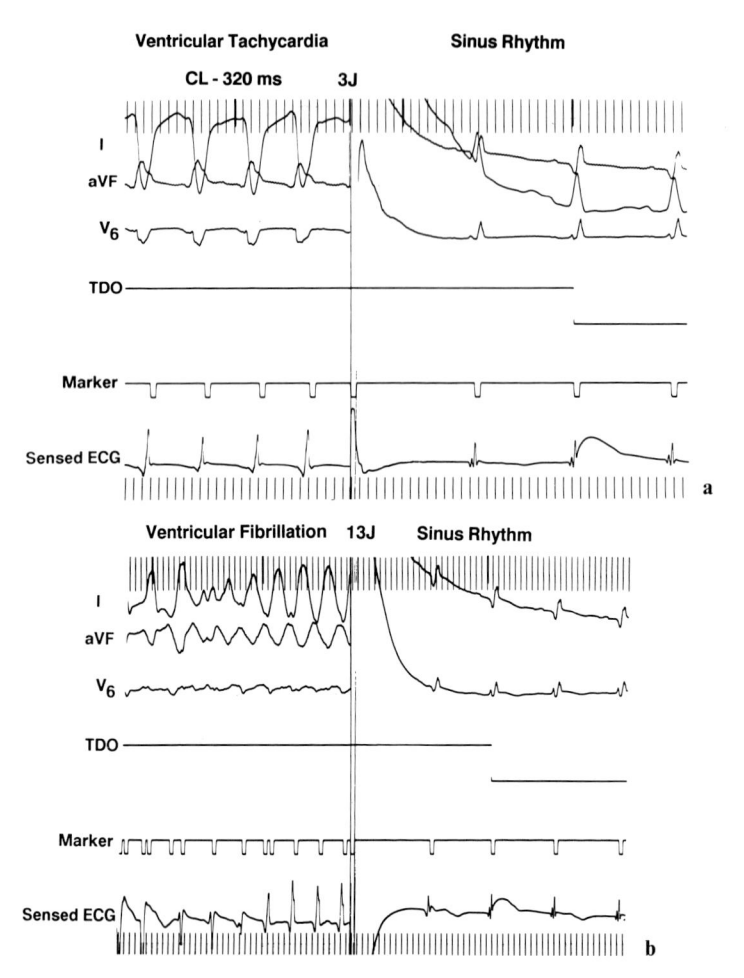

Fig. 4a, b. Implantation of a programmable pacemaker-cardioverter-defibrillator. Threshold testing for ventricular tachycardia and ventricular fibrillation is performed. **a** Induced ventricular tachycardia is cardioverted with a 3-J shock delivered using two patch electrodes. TDO, ventricular tachycardia detector output; ECG, electrocardiogram; CL, cycle length. **b** Induced ventricular fibrillation in the same patient as in **a** is now converted with a 13-J shock. Abbreviations as in **a**

systems. We and others have demonstrated that defibrillation thresholds can be reduced by the use of asymmetric biphasic waveform shocks [42]. These asymmetric biphasic waveform shocks can reduce the capacitor/battery requirements for an implantable pulse generator. Should clinical trials validate reduction in defibrillation threshold, significant reduction in pulse generator size can be expected. The use of a generic lead system for pacing, sensing, and endocardial defibrillation using standard dual chamber implant techniques is being developed. Such an approach would provide cardioversion defibrillation therapy as an extension of current pacing techniques.

It is readily conceivable that implantable cardioverter-defibrillators will provide a serious therapeutic option for patients with congestive heart failure and sustained VT or ventricular fibrillation. Implantation of endocardial lead systems will reduce implant morbidity and mortality to acceptable levels. Should comparable efficacy to epicardial defibrillation lead systems be demonstrated, this approach will provide antiarrhythmic efficacy of an exceedingly high degree. Use of multiprogrammable devices and availability of multiple electrical therapies will provide for treatment of both bradycardias and tachycardias in these patients. This should permit this nonpharmacologic approach to be used in conjunction with aggressive management techniques for congestive heart failure. Implant of epicardial lead system may be restricted in the future to patients undergoing major cardiac surgical procedures for their congestive heart failure. Implantable cardioverter-defibrillator therapy would be applicable to patients with paroxysmal ventricular tachycardia for ventricular fibrillation, irrespective of rate, morphology or underlying heart disease. It can be expected to be used in conjunction with antiarrhythmic drug therapy or ablation techniques. It is inapplicable to patients with incessant or frequent VT ventricular fibrillation. It will also be available as alternative therapy for patients who are only partially or inadequately controlled by drug or ablation therapy. These nonpharmacologic approaches for the treatment of sustained ventricular tachyarrhythmias will offer an important option to current pharmacologic approaches, particularly in patients with significant left ventricular dysfunction and congestive heart failure.

References

1. An H, Saksena S, Janssen M, Osypka P (1989) Radiofrequency ablation of ventricular myocardium using active fixation and passive contact catheter delivery systems. Am Heart J 118:69
2. Bach SM, Barstad J, Harper N et al. (1989) Initial clinical experience: Endotak-implantable transvenous defibrillator system. J Am Coll Cardiol 13:65A
3. Borggrefe M, Budde T, Martinez-Rubio A et al. (1988) Radiofrequency catheter ablation for drug resistant supraventricular tachycardia. Circulation 78 [Suppl II]:II-305
4. Borggrefe M, Podczeck A, Ostermeyer J et al. (1987) Long term results of electrophysiologically guided tachycardia surgery in ventricular tachyarrhythmias. A collaborative report on 665 patients. In: Breithardt G, Borggrefe M, Zipes DP (eds) Non-pharmacological therapy of tachyarrhythmias. Futura, Mount Kisco, p 109
5. Branyas NA, Cain ME, Cassidy DM (1989) Transmural ventricular activation during consecutive cycles of sustained ventricular tachycardia. J Am Coll Cardiol 13:167A
6. Calvo RA, Saksena S, Pantopoulos D (1988) Sequential transvenous pacing and shock therapy for termination of sustained ventricular tachycardia. Am Heart J 115:569
7. Camm AJ, Ward DE, Spurell RAJ et al. (1980) Cryothermal mapping and cryoablation in the treatment of refractory cardiac arrhythmias. Circulation 62:67
8. CASS principal investigators and their associates (1983) Coronary artery surgery study (CASS): A randomized trial of coronary artery bypass surgery survival data. Circulation 68:939
9. Ciccone JM, Saksena S, Shah Y et al. (1985) A prospective, randomized study of the clinical efficacy and safety of transvenous cardioversion for ventricular tachycardia termination. Circulation 71:571

10. DePaola AAV, Horowitz LN, Morganroth J, Senior S, Spielman SR, Greenspan AM, Kay HR (1987) Influence of left ventricular dysfunction on flecainide therapy. J Am Coll Cardiol 9:163
11. Downar E, Mickleborough LL, Harris L et al. (1986) Mapping of endocardial activation during ventricular tachycardia – a "closed heart" procedure. J Am Coll Cardiol 7:234
12. ESVEM Investigators (1989) The ESVEM trial: electrophysiologic study versus electrocardiographic monitoring for selection of antiarrhythmic therapy of ventricular tachyarrhythmias. Circulation 79:1354
13. Evans GT Jr, Scheinman MM (1987) The percutaneous cardiac mapping and ablation registry: summary of results. PACE 10:1395
14. Fisher JD, Kim SG, Matos JA et al. (1983) Comparative effectiveness of pacing techniques for termination of well-tolerated sustained ventricular tachycardia. PACE 6:915
15. Follansbee WP, Michelson EL, Morganroth J (1980) Nonsustained ventricular tachycardia in ambulatory patients: characteristics and association with sudden cardiac death. Ann Intern Med 92:741
16. Gallagher JJ, Svenson RH, Kasell JH et al. (1982) Catheter technique for closed chest ablation of the atrioventricular conduction system. A therapeutic alternative for the treatment of refractory supraventricular tachycardia. N Engl J Med 306:194
17. Huang SK, Bharati S, Graham AR et al. (1987) Closed chest catheter desiccation of the atrioventricular junction using radiofrequency energy – a new method of catheter ablation. J Am Coll Cardiol 9:349
18. Josephson ME, Horowitz LN, Farshid A et al. (1978) Recurrent sustained ventricular tachycardia. 2. Endocardial mapping. Circulation 57:440
19. Josephson ME, Harken AH, Horowitz LN (1979) Endocardial excision: a new surgical technique for the treatment of recurrent ventricular tachycardia. Circulation 60:1430
20. Lavery S, Saksena S (1987) Management of refractory sustained ventricular tachycardia with amiodarone: a reappraisal. Am Heart J 113:49
21. Lindsay BD, Saksena S, Rothbart ST et al. (1987) Prospective evaluation of a sequential pacing and high-energy bidirectional shock algorithm for transvenous cardioversion in patients with ventricular tachycardia. Circulation 76:601
22. Miller JM, Kienzle MG, Harken AH et al. (1984) Subendocardial resection for ventricular tachycardia: predictors of surgical success. Circulation 70:624
23. Milrinone Multicenter Trial Group (1989) A comparison of oral milrinone, digoxin, and their combination in the treatment of patients with chronic heart failure. N Engl J Med 320:677
24. Mirowski M, Reid PR, Mower MM et al. (1980) Termination of malignant ventricular arrhythmias with an implanted automatic defibrillator in human beings. N Engl J Med 303:322
25. Packer M (1985) Sudden unexpected death in patients with congestive heart failure: a second frontier. Circulation 72:681
26. Saksena S (1989) Catheter ablation of tachycardias with laser energy: issues and answers. PACE 12:196
27. Saksena S, An HL (1990) Clinical efficacy of dual electrode systems for endocardial cardioversion of ventricular tachycardia: a prospective randomized crossover trial. Am Heart J 119:15
28. Saksena S, Calvo R (1985) Transvenous cardioversion and defibrillation of ventricular tachyarrhythmias: current status and future directions. PAGE 8:715
29. Saksena S, Gadhoke A (1986) Laser therapy for tachyarrhythmias: a new frontier. PACE 9:531
30. Saksena S, Gielchinsky I (1988) Intraoperative selection of laser ablation site in patients with sustained ventricular tachycardia. PACE 11:528
31. Saksena S, Parsonnet V (1988) Implantation of a cardioverter/defibrillator without thoracotomy using a triple electrode system. JAMA 259:69
32. Saksena S, Chandran P, Shah Y et al. (1985) Comparative efficacy of transvenous cardioversion and pacing in patients with sustained ventricular tachycardia: a prospective randomized crossover study. Circulation 72:153

33. Saksena S, Ciccone J, Chandran P et al. (1986) Laser ablation of normal and diseased human ventricle. Am Heart J 112:52
34. Saksena S, Hussain SM, Wasty N et al. (1986) Long-term efficacy of subendocardial resection in refractory ventricular tachycardia: relationship to site of arrhythmia origin. Ann Thorac Surg 42:685
35. Saksena S, Calvo RA, Pantopoulos D et al. (1987) A prospective evaluation of single and dual current pathways for transvenous cardioversion in rapid ventricular tachycardia. PACE 10:1130
36. Saksena S, Hussain SM, Gielchinsky I et al. (1987) Intraoperative mapping-guided argon laser ablation of malignant ventricular tachycardia. Am J Cardiol 59:78
37. Saksena S, Lindsay BD, Parsonnet V (1987) Development of future implantable cardioverters and defibrillators. PACE 10:1342
38. Saksena S, Pantopoulos D, Hussain SM et al. (1987) Mechanisms of ventricular tachycardia termination and acceleration during transvenous cardioversion as determined by cardiac mapping in man. Am Heart J 113:1495
39. Saksena S, Tarjan PP, Bharati S et al. (1987) Low energy transvenous ablation of the atrioventricular conduction system using a suction electrode catheter. Circulation 76:394
40. Saksena S, Hussain SM, Gielchinsky I (1988) Surgical ablation of tachyarrhythmias: reflections for the third decade (editorial). PACE 11:103
41. Saksena S, Gielchinsky I, Tullo NG (1989) Argon laser ablation of malignant ventricular tachycardia associated with coronary artery disease. Am J Cardiol 64:1298
42. Saksena S, Scott S, Accorti P et al. (1989) Improved pacing and internal defibrillation using a porous electrode catheter with biphasic unidirectional and bidirectional shocks. PACE 12(I):663
43. Saksena S, Tullo NG, Krol RB et al. (1989) Initial clinical experience with endocardial defibrillation using an implantable cardioverter/defibrillator with a triple electrode system. Arch Intern Med 149:2333
44. Scheinman MM, Morady F, Hess DS et al. (1982) Catheter induced ablation of the atrioventricular junction to control refractory supraventricular arrhythmias. JAMA 248:851
45. Thomas A, Moser SA, Smutka ML et al. (1988) Implantable defibrillation: eight year clinical experience. PACE 11:2053
46. Tullo NG, An H, Saksena S (1989) Ablation using radiofrequency current and low energy D.C. shocks. In: Saksena S, Goldschlager N (eds) Textbook of electrical therapy for cardiac arrhythmias. Saunders, Philadelphia
47. Vedel J, Frank R, Fontaine G et al. (1979) Bloc auriculo-ventriculaire intra-Hisien definitif induit au cours d'une exploration endoventriculaire droite. Arch Mal Coeur 72:107
48. Veltri EP, Reid PR, Platia EV, Griffith LSC (1985) Amiodarone in the treatment of life-threatening ventricular tachycardia: role of Holter monitoring in predicting long-term clinical efficacy. J Am Coll Cardiol 6:806
49. Warin JF, Hassaguerre M, Lemetayer P et al. (1988) Catheter ablation of accessory pathways with a direct approach. Circulation 78:800
50. Wilber DJ, Garan H, Finkelstein D et al. (1988) Out of hospital cardiac arrest: use of electrophysiologic testing in the prediction of long-term outcome. N Engl J Med 38:19
51. Zipes DP, Jackman WM, Heger JJ (1982) Clinical transvenous cardioversion of recurrent life-threatening tachyarrhythmias: low energy synchronized cardioversion of ventricular tachycardia and termination of ventricular fibrillation in patients using a catheter electrode. Am Heart J 103:789

Role of Antiarrhythmic Drug Therapy in Patients with Congestive Heart Failure

R. L. Woosley

The presence of arrhythmias in patients with congestive heart failure (CHF) is an independent risk factor for sudden death, and approximately 50% of deaths in patients with CHF can be characterized as sudden. The incidence of sudden arrhythmic death in patients with CHF is difficult to ascertain but is probably between 30% and 50% per year [1–3]. Therefore, reduction of the risk of sudden cardiac death in patients with CHF is a desirable clinical goal. Three reports have been made on the effects of antiarrhythmic drugs on mortality in patients with CHF. Chakko and Gheorghiade [1] described their uncontrolled retrospective experience with antiarrhythmic drugs in 43 patients and found no difference in outcome (Fig. 1). Subsequently, Parmley and Chatterjee [2] reported on a subgroup of patients with CHF, who were in studies originally designed to evaluate new inotropic drugs. Figure 2 demonstrates the differences in outcome depending on whether antiarrhythmic drugs were prescribed or not. This uncontrolled experience found lower mortality in those patients given quinidine, procainamide, or amiodarone and led the authors to call for a prospective and randomized trial to address the true value of antiarrhythmic drugs in such patients. Nicklas and his colleagues [3] at Michigan have reported in abstract form their experience in a prospective randomized evaluation of 100 patients treated with low dose amiodarone or placebo. Although this was a small study and lacked adequate power to detect any significant effect, there was no evidence of benefit from amiodarone (see Table 1). Therefore, there are conflicting data in the literature and no well-designed prospective study exists with adequate power to determine the value of antiarrhythmic drugs in this population.

In order to put the question of therapy in this population in perspective, one might ask if antiarrhythmic drugs are effective in other populations. For high risk patients, those who have been resuscitated from sudden death or have recurrent ventricular tachycardia (VT), there is general consensus that carefully selected antiarrhythmic drugs, which prevent induction of the clinical arrhythmia by programmed ventricular stimulation, will prevent arrhythmia recurrence or sud-

Table 1. Survival in patients on amiodarone. (From Nicklas et al. [3])

	6 months survival	1 year survival
Placebo	87%	72%
Amiodarone	84%	75%

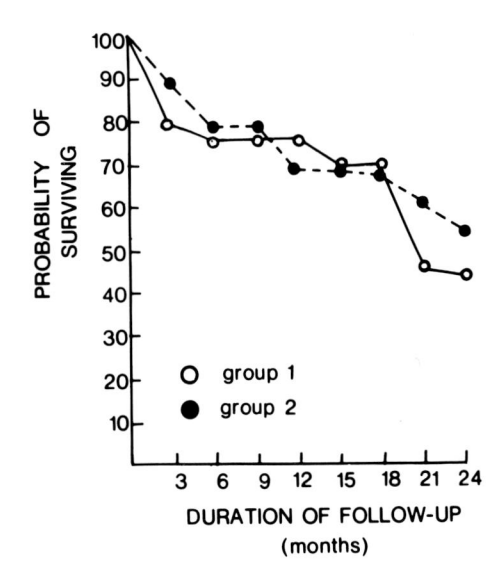

Fig. 1. Survival curves in the group receiving antiarrhythmic drug therapy (*open circle*) and the group not receiving antiarrhythmic drug therapy (*closed circle*). Based on Chakko and Gheorghiade [1]

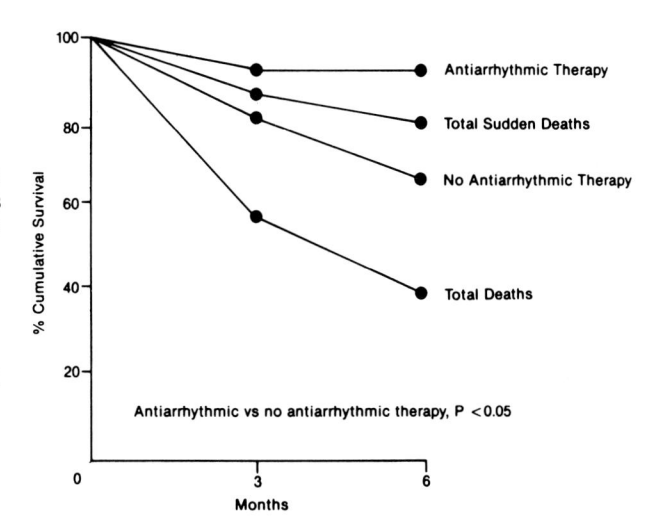

Fig. 2. Incidence of sudden death was lower in patients with severe congestive heart failure and complex ventricular arrhythmias who were receiving newer inotropic vasodilator agents plus antiarrhythmic therapy, than in those who did not receive antiarrhythmic drugs. Based on Parmley and Chatterjee [2]

den death. However, this is difficult to prove because there are no controlled trials. All available reports indicate that those patients who appear to have a good clinical response (determined either by programmed ventricular stimulation or noninvasive evaluation) have a lower rate of arrhythmia recurrence or sudden death. However, since patients with severe heart disease and arrhythmias are more refractory to therapy [4], response to therapy may select a population with a lower inherent risk for sudden death or arrhythmia recurrence. With the availability of the automatic internal cardioverter/defibrillator (AICD), it may soon be possible to perform randomized placebo-controlled trials to address the value of these drugs in this high risk population.

At the other end of the spectrum are patients with asymptomatic arrhythmias and no known structural heart disease. Antiarrhythmic therapy is clearly not indicated for these patients, who are at low risk of sudden death [5]. In the middle of the spectrum are the largest number of patients: those with ventricular arrhythmias and structural heart disease (usually postmyocardial infarction). These patients have prognostically significant arrhythmias, i.e., factors predicting a higher risk of sudden death. The Cardiac Arrhythmia Suppression Trial (CAST) tested the hypothesis that suppression of asymptomatic ventricular arrhythmias in patients who have previously had myocardial infarction and whose ventricular function is impaired would reduce the incidence of sudden death [6]. The driving force for this study was the availability of drugs capable of suppressing ventricular arrhythmias and their widespread prescription by cardiologists for this purpose. A survey in 1984 by Vlay [7] found that 70–90% of cardiologists at 65 academic centers prescribed antiarrhythmic drugs for these patients. To fully understand the results of CAST and its implication for patients with arrhythmias and CHF, it is essential to review the objectives and design of the study.

CAST was designed to mimic, as closely as possible, the practice of cardiology in the 1980's. It had a difficult task: to test an important hypothesis using a controlled clinical trial protocol. Since the early 1980's it has been common practice to perform a 24-h ambulatory ECG recording (AECG) in patients recovering from myocardial infarction. Repeat AECGs were usually performed to be certain that the patient's rhythm has improved. Based on data from a large number of postinfarction trials [8], patients with reduced ventricular function who are also found on AECG to have high frequency ventricular arrhythmias or, particularly, runs of VT are considered to be at higher risk of sudden death. These patients have been treated aggressively, commonly with quinidine, procainamide, disopyramide, tocainide, or mexiletine. Recently they have even been enrolled in trials in which programmed ventricular stimulation is used to evaluate their propensity to sustained ventricular tachyarrhythmias [9]. These patients are often classified as having "potentially malignant" ventricular arrhythmias [10], a term that encourages aggressive therapy. However, this is an especially unsatisfactory term because it includes such a wide spectrum of patients, ranging from those postmyocardial infarction patients with normal ventricular function and rare premature ventricular depolarizations (PVDs) to those with severe ventricular dysfunction and nonsustained VT. The annual incidence of sudden death may vary from 2% in the former group to up to 50% in the latter [8]. Clearly, there has been a need for research to help physicians develop a sound approach for the proper treatment of these patients.

Before CAST, the National Institutes of Health (NIH) sponsored a feasibility trial, the Cardiac Arrhythmia Pilot Study (CAPS) [4]. CAPS enrolled 502 patients in a placebo-controlled comparison of four drugs chosen for their potential to suppress ambient ventricular arrhythmia without causing intolerable side effects. CAPS found that encainide and flecainide were the most effective in suppressing PVDs, with moricizine being slightly less effective. All three were well-tolerated, with the incidence of side effects being not significantly different from placebo. Importantly, the incidence of arrhythmia aggravation and death was also low and indistinguishable from that in the placebo group. However, the overall incidence of CHF was high in each of the five treatment arms, and the group randomized to flecainide had the highest incidence. This was not statistically significant, but because of simultaneous reports of new and worsened heart failure with flecainide, the observation was considered in the design of CAST. The major conclusions from CAPS were that it was feasible (1) to enroll patients with ventricular arrhythmias after myocardial infarction, (2) to effectively suppress their arrhythmias for at least 1 year, and (3) to use AECG to evaluate the degree of arrhythmia suppression. Therefore, in 1987 the NIH chose 23 sites in the U.S., three in Canada and one in Sweden to perform CAST. Based on an expected incidence of sudden death of 11% over 3 years, it was estimated that 4400 patients would be required to detect a 30% reduction in sudden cardiac death. A Data and Safety Monitoring Board (DSMB) was chosen to review the progress and instructed to recommend halting the trial if (1) benefit was proven, (2) harm was detected, or (3) there was no chance that a beneficial effect could be found within the established study period.

The design of the study is shown in Fig. 3 and the inclusion and exclusion criteria are listed in Table 2. Because the incidence of sudden death decreases after the first 3 months following myocardial infarction [8], the entry criteria demanded a greater degree of left ventricular dysfunction after that time in order to exclude patients at low risk for sudden death. Patients who met entry criteria and agreed to participate entered an open label titration phase that was similar to usual clinical practice. It differed only in that the order of drug selection was randomized and influenced by the patients' ventricular function. Those with an ejection fraction of at least 30% were randomized to one of two arms which included encainide or flecainide, the two drugs in CAPS which were most effective in

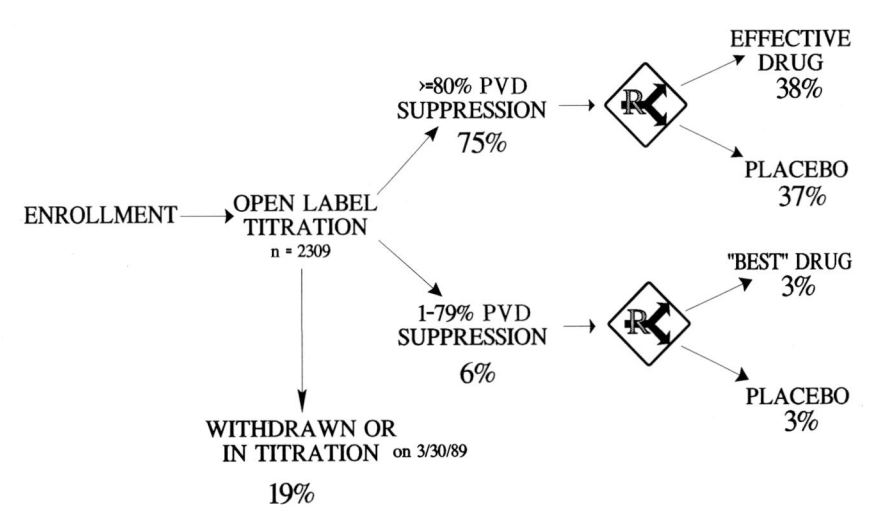

Fig. 3. CAST study design. After enrollment, drug and dose selection was performed in an unblinded phase in which 81% of patients were identified as responders to encainide, flecainide, or moricizine (75% of total patients) and those with partial suppression (6% of patients). Both of these groups were separately randomized (*R symbol*) to remain on therapy or to receive a placebo in the double blind phase of the study. "Best" drug refers to the drug which produced the greatest degree of partial suppression without causing side effects

Table 2. Major inclusion and exclusion criteria for CAST

Inclusion	6 days to 2 years after myocardial infarction
	≥ 6 PVDs/h on an 18–24 h ambulatory ECG
	Reduced ventricular function (ejection fraction)
	ejection fraction ≤ 0.55 6–90 days after MI
	ejection fraction ≤ 0.40 90 days–2 years after MI
Exclusion	Severely symptomatic arrhythmias
	Age > 79 years
	VT > 14 beats
	Other life-threatening conditions

suppressing premature ventricular depolarizations (PVD). Those with an ejection fraction of less than 30% were randomized to receive either encainide or moricizine because of the perceived increased risk of CHF with flecainide. Those patients whose ventricular ectopy is suppressed by greater than 80% and who have at least 90% suppression of runs of VT were randomized to remain on active drug therapy or to receive a placebo. These 1727 patients were in the main treatment arm of the study, which included approximately 75% of those who began titration. A smaller number of patients had partial suppression and entered a substudy, in which they were also randomized to drug or placebo.

The study was interrupted early when the DSMB asked the investigators to remove two of the drugs from the study because of increased deaths during the randomized period of follow-up. The drug code was broken and it was found that the excess mortality was seen with only two of the drugs, encainide and flecainide. A small number of subjects were being followed in the moricizine arm and there was no evidence of harm in this group. Therefore, the DSMB recommended that the study continue with moricizine and (because of a high incidence of death in the open label phase) be redesigned to include a placebo period in the drug titration phase. Figure 4 demonstrates the increased incidence of sudden death and total mortality in the group treated with encainide or flecainide.

Table 3 lists the characteristics of the CAST patients who were in the encainide or flecainide arms of the study. As can be seen, this is a population that most cardiologists would have considered to be at high risk for sudden death and therefore require antiarrhythmic therapy. However, in this case, mortality in the placebo arm was much lower than expected and less than that seen in patients who received either of the two drugs that suppressed arrhythmias.

What, then, should be recommended for the large number of patients with a history of CHF who also have asymptomatic ventricular arrhythmias? The data available indicate that effective therapy to control the patient's heart failure will improve the quality of life and that therapy with angiotensin-converting enzyme inhibitors will decrease mortality [11]. Symptomatic CHF was not an enrollment criterion for CAST, but all patients had some evidence of ventricular dysfunction: 50% of the patients had an ejection fraction less than 0.4 and 15% had an ejection fraction less than 0.3. The increased mortality was common to all groups in CAST, including those with the lowest ejection fraction, and is likely to be seen in patients with a history of CHF and asymptomatic ventricular arrhythmias.

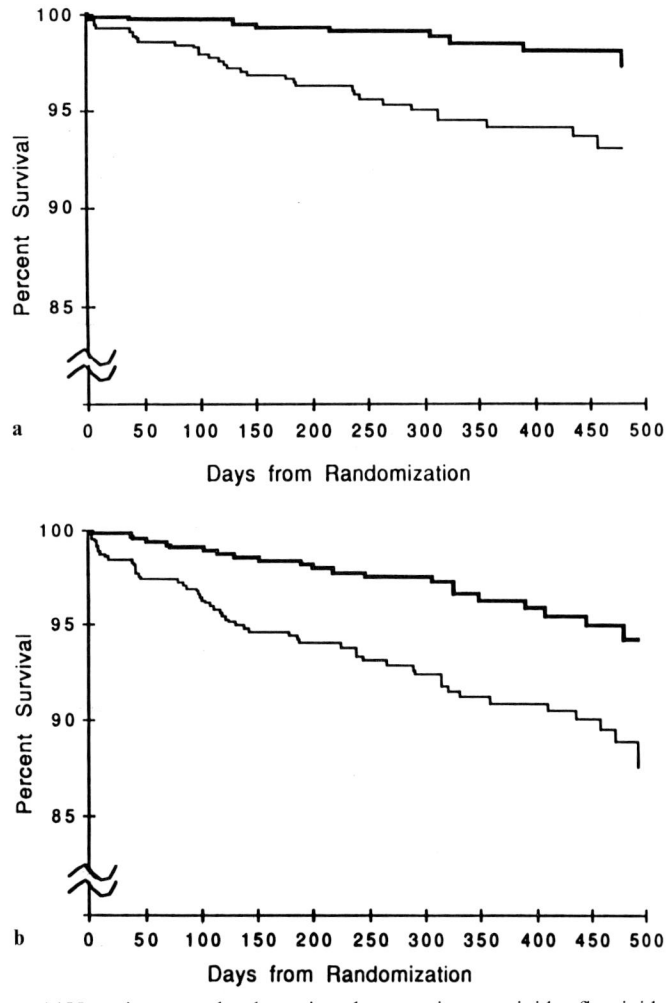

Fig. 4a, b. Survival among 1455 patients randomly assigned to receive encainide, flecainide ($n=730$; *thin line*), or matching placebo ($n=725$; *thick line*). **a** The cause of death was arrhythmia or cardiac arrest ($p=0.0006$). **b** Based on data for all causes of death ($p=0.0003$). The nominal *p* values in **a** and **b** were based on a traditional two-sided log-rank test adjusted for multiple groups. (From [6] with permission)

Therefore, the data from CAST and the limited data from other trials with patients with CHF [1–3] do not support the use of the local anesthetic class of antiarrhythmic drugs in these patients and actually suggests that some may be contraindicated. Until a clinical trial has been performed with such patients, the use of antiarrhythmic drugs must be considered of unproven benefit. This is another clinical problem for which the words of Sherlock Holmes best describe our current state of knowledge: "I have no data yet. It is capital mistake to theorize before one has data. One insensibly begins to twist facts to suit the theories instead of theories to suit the facts" [12].

Table 3. Baseline characteristics of 1455 patients randomized to encainide or flecainide or matching placebo. (Adapted from [6] with permission)

	Encainide/Flecainide	Placebo
Canadian angina class		
no angina	81.4%	80.7%
I	8.7%	9.1%
II	7.7%	8.6%
III	2.3%	1.6%
Smoking		
present	39.8%	39.1%
former	41.4%	40.8%
never	18.8%	20.1%
MI to Holter ≥ 90 days	21.4%	21.9%
Baseline ECG		
PR interval (s)	0.17 (±0.03)	0.17 (±0.03)
QRS duration (s)	0.09 (±0.02)	0.09 (±0.02)
QT interval (s), uncorrected	0.39 (±0.04)	0.39 (±0.04)
Atrial fibrillation or flutter	2.0%	1.3%
Left ventricular hypertrophy	4.7%	2.7%
Paced	0.4%	0.3%
Baseline holter		
PVD/h	127 (±254)	128 (±249)
≤10	15.1%	16.2%
10.1 – 50	39.8%	40.7%
50.1 – 100	17.6%	15.8%
≥100	27.5%	27.3%
VT runs (≥120 bpm)/24 h		
none	78.8%	79.9%
1	10.7%	11.4%
2–5	6.2%	5.2%
≥6	4.3%	3.5%
Atrial fibrillation of flutter	3.5%	2.6%
Permanent pacemaker	1.1%	1.7%
LBBB	1.8%	1.7%
Baseline physical exam		
Sitting heart rate	74 (±13)	73 (±13)
Systolic blood pressure	126 (±18)	125 (±18)
Diastolic blood pressure	77 (±11)	76 (±10)
Concurrent drugs at baseline		
Beta blocker	30.4%	33.1%
Calcium entry blocker	52.3%	49.3%
Digitalis	21.2%	18.5%

References

1. Chakko CS, Gheorghiade M (1985) Ventricular arrhythmias in severe heart failure: incidence, significance, and effectiveness of antiarrhythmic therapy. Am Heart J 109:497–504
2. Parmley WW, Chatterjee K (1986) Congestive heart failure and arrhythmias: an overview. Am J Cardiol 57:34b–37b

3. Nicklas JM, Mickelson JK, Das SK, Morady F, Schork MA, Pitt B (1988) Prospective, randomized, double-blind, placebo-controlled trial of low dose amiodarone in patients with severe heart failure and frequent ventricular ectopy. Circulation 78(4):II-27A
4. Cardiac Arrhythmia Pilot Study (CAPS) Investigators (1988) Effects of encainide, flecainide, imipramine and moricizine on ventricular arrhythmias during the year after acute myocardial infarction: the CAPS. Am J Cardiol 61:501–509
5. Kennedy HL, Whitlock JA, Sprague MK et al. (1985) Long-term follow-up of asymptomatic healthy subjects with frequent and complex ventricular ectopy. N Engl J Med 312:193–197
6. Cardiac Arrhythmia Suppression Trial (CAST) Investigators (1989) Preliminary report: effect of encainide and flecainide on mortality in a randomized trial of arrhythmia suppression after myocardial infarction. N Engl J Med 321:406–412
7. Vlay SC (1985) How the university cardiologist treats ventricular premature beats: a nationwide survey of 65 university medical centers. Am Heart J 110:904–912
8. Bigger JT Jr (1986) Relation between left ventricular dysfunction and ventricular arrhythmias after myocardial infarction. Am J Cardiol 57:8B–14B
9. Klein SW, Machell C (1989) Use of electrophysiologic testing in patients with nonsustained ventricular tachycardia: prognostic and therapeutic implications. Am J Cardiol 14:155–161
10. Morganroth J (1984) Premature ventricular complexes. Diagnosis and indications for therapy. JAMA 252:673–676
11. Consensus Trial Study Group (1987) Effects of enalapril on mortality in severe congestive failure. Results of the Cooperative North Scandinavian Enalapril Survival Study. N Engl J Med 316(23):1429–1435
12. Conan Doyle A (1976) A scandal in Bohemia. In: The illustrated Sherlock Holmes treasury. The adventures of Sherlock Holmes. Crown, New York

III Prognosis

Obtaining Reliable Information from Randomized Controlled Trials in Congestive Heart Failure and Left Ventricular Dysfunction

S. YUSUF

Introduction

Chronic congestive heart failure (CHF) is a syndrome that is the end result of a number of different kinds of cardiac damage and compensatory mechanisms resulting in a variable prognosis. Patients usually have a high mortality rate, a high rate of morbid complications, and multiple severe symptoms. The high rates of morbidity and symptoms lead to limitations in daily activities and poor quality of life. The aim of therapy in such patients should therefore be not only the amelioration of symptoms and signs of CHF but also the prevention of morbidity, improvement in quality of life, and prolongation of survival. Because the clinical course in a particular patient is highly variable and unpredictable, the effect of a therapy can be reliably evaluated only if all sources of errors in this evaluation are minimized. In general, errors can be classified into those due to systematic biases and those due to random errors. In order to avoid a variety of systematic biases randomized double-blind controlled trials are essential. Such studies avoid biases in patient allocation, minimize imbalances at entry use of other therapy, and avoid biases in endpoint ascertainment. In this chapter, I will discuss the following issues:

1. The likely size of effect with currently available interventions.
2. Why randomized trials are essential in heart failure.
3. Why some of the trials should be much larger than those that have been conducted.
4. How some of the currently employed methods of analysis and reporting can be biased and can lead to misleading conclusions.
5. Why one may not be able to extrapolate from the effect of a particular agent on surrogate endpoints (such as exercise tolerance) to clinically relevant outcomes such as survival or morbidity.
6. How the framework of the trials and the data that are collected systematically provide an opportunity to learn more about the clinical course of patients with heart failure.
7. Examples of some large studies that are in progress.

Why Are Moderate Effects on Major Endpoints Generally more Plausible than Large Ones?

If any widely practicable intervention had a very large effect, e.g., a cure for most patients in a common condition such as heart failure with high mortality, then whether or nor randomized trials are conducted, these huge gains by the therapy are likely to be identified more or less reliably by simple clinical observation, by historically controlled comparisons, or by a variety of other informal or semiformal nonrandomized methods. Such methods may well suffer from moderate biases, but despite their deficiencies they may eventually yield a reliable consensus. Although large therapeutic improvements may be accepted more rapidly if the stringent test of a randomized controlled study is undertaken, they will probably eventually gain acceptance anyway. So, if there remains some controversy about the efficacy of any widely practicable treatment, its effects on major endpoints may well be either nil, or moderate rather than large. This does not necessarily apply to its effects on various nonclinical surrogate endpoints, e.g., various measures of the extent or progress of the disease. For example, it is not difficult to demonstrate that ventricular arrythmia may be reduced with an antiarrhythmic agent. However for other endpoints such as exercise tolerance or changes in left ventricular function, the benefits of various treatments, especially during long-term therapy, have been relatively modest. Furthermore, it is extremely difficult to prevent (or substantially delay) a large proportion of deaths, especially in patients who have already sustained extensive cardiac damage. Indirect support for this conclusion comes from many sources, including (a) the previous few decades of disappointingly slow progress in the treatment of patients with heart failure; (b) the heterogeneity of the disease, as evidenced by the unpredictability of survival duration even when apparently similar patients are compared with each other; (c) the variety of different mechanisms that can, in principle, lead to death, only one of which may be appreciably influenced by one particular therapy; and (d) experience with many earlier trials, review of which (Table 1) suggests that the true risk reductions being studied were probably only of the order of 15%, 20%, or 25% rather than for example 40%, 50%, or 60% [1].

Points b, c, and d perhaps deserve some expansion and illustration. First, although several important prognostic features can be identified in patients with heart failure, the exact mechanism(s) by which they are related to a particular patient's outcome is unclear. For example, we often do not know why one heart failure patient with a particular complication such as ventricular tachycardia may live for several years whereas another may die tomorrow. In other words, even within subgroups of patients who are, by currently available criteria, fairly similar to each other, there is considerable heterogeneity of outcome, i.e., the outcome may be dictated chiefly by unknown or unmeasured features (and hence, perhaps, by mechanisms that we do not deliberately affect).

Secondly, we may know of several different mechanisms that could lead to death, and current drug treatments are usually aimed at modifying only one or two of these at a time. For example, elevated catecholamines, elevated renin, ischemia, peripheral vascular constriction, cardiac muscle wall stress, arrhythmi-

Table 1. "Plausible" risk reductions in mortality with various treatments in patients with heart failure

Treatment	Number of trials	Approximate number of patients	Approximate mortality reduction (% ±SE)[a]
Based on studies with mostly 3- to 6-month follow-up			
Direct-acting vasodilators	5	180	+38% (±30%)
ACE inhibitors	9	900	−30% (±14%)
Alpha-blockers	8	250	0% (±20%)
Beta-blockers	4	130	−25% (±30%)
Inotropic agents (nondigitalis)	5	1000	+90% (±30%)
Digitalis	3	600	very limited data
Based on studies with about 6-month to 1-year follow-up			
ACE inhibitors	2	450	−20% (±11%)
Based on studies with more than 1-year follow-up			
Alpha-blockers	1	450	0% (±15%)
Hydralazine + nitrates	1	450	−25% (±14%)

[a] These are estimates based upon the pooled data of various small randomized trials. The primary aim of most trials was to assess the effect of treatment on a surrogate endpoint such as exercise capacity. Most of these estimates have fairly large standard errors and consequently the true effect with almost all the interventions are subject to considerable uncertainty. A − sign indicates a reduction in mortality. A + sign indicates an increase in mortality.

as, changes in preload and afterload, and contractile stress, are each associated with somewhat different mechanisms by which prognosis could be worsened. Although these mechanisms are unlikely to be of equal importance, there are so many of them that it might be unrealistic to expect modification of any single factor by a particular intervention to reduce mortality by a large proportion (e.g., by more than 30%) although it may be realistic to hope for some more moderate benefits (e.g., 10% or 20%). Finally, returning to the (rather sobering) data in Table 1, it appears that few interventions have been reliably assessed. Where a reasonable amount of information is available, the mortality reduction suggested by the pooled data for that intervention is only moderate (e.g., 20%–30%). Indeed, even the available data on the more promising agents such as ACE inhibitors are restricted to very select patients followed for relatively short periods.

If indeed, with many currently available agents, only moderate reductions in mortality are plausible, how worthwhile might such effects be, if they could be reliably detected? To some clinicians, reducing the risk of death heart failure from 15 per 100 to 12 per 100 treated patients for a year may not seem particularly worthwhile, and indeed if such a reduction were achievable only at the expense of prolonged treatment by an expensive or toxic agent, this might well be an appropriate view. On the other hand, since death due to heart failure is common, a simple, widely practicable treatment with acceptable side effects, that reduced the risk of death by perhaps 10%–20% (i.e., from 15% dead to 13.5% or 12%) could, on a national or international scale, have substantial public health implications and might, for example, substantially delay several tens of thousands of deaths per year in the United States alone. These absolute gains are substantial (and might, indeed, considerably exceed the numbers of lives that could hypothetically be saved by a simple cure for all patients with some less common disease such as acute myeloid leukemia).

Randomized Trials Are Essential for Unbiased Evaluation of Therapy

It is obvious to all clinicians who treat patients with heart failure that these patients often present with a wide spectrum of signs and symptoms. The etiology of the disease is variable. The extent and type of ventricular dysfunction differ; the types and degree of compensatory neurohumoral, renal and other reflex mechanisms are heterogenous. It is therefore not surprising that despite very detailed characterization of a patient's status his or her prognosis cannot be accurately predicted, partly because we are unaware of many of the important prognostic features and partly because of uncertainty regarding the precise influence of a particular factor on outcome. This realization has two important implications. First, if one tries to constitute two groups of patients that are supposedly "matched" by all known measures (i.e., two nonrandomized groups), one would still not be surprised if the outcomes in the two groups differed simply by chance. Second, in studies in which a treatment is to be evaluated, trying to match patients who are prescribed a particular drug (because of the severity of their condition) with those who were not almost always leads to systematic selection biases. Even if we were able to measure every *known* relevant factor, statistical adjustments are generally inadequate and cannot assure that patients who have received the new drug and those who did not, can be matched sufficiently. Therefore for almost all nonrandomized estimates, one cannot be certain that any observed differences are due to a treatment effect or simply to patient selection. Since the degree of benefit from most treatments in heart failure is likely to be modest (such as improvement in exercise tolerance by 10% or 20%, or reduction in long-term mortality and morbidity by 10%, 15%, or 20%) even the moderate biases and errors inherent in methods which use nonrandomized controls should be avoided.

Control of the various biases and errors described above is best accomplished through randomization of patients to the various study groups. In general, randomization avoids biases in the assignment of who does and does not receive therapy and consequently tends to result in groups similar in all measured (and likely all unmeasured) factors, at the start of the study. Therefore any subsequent change in clinical condition can be presumed to be related to the intervention as distinguished from "natural" changes that occur due to patients spontaneously getting better or worse. Because randomization tends to ensure equalization of all relevant factors, it no longer becomes necessary to collect a lot of data on each patient. Instead, only few key variables that are needed to describe the population or those relevant to performing important subgroup analyses are required at baseline, in addition to data on compliance and the outcome(s) of interest. Consequently studies that involve randomized comparisons can be conducted at far lower costs than similar, studies involving nonrandomized groups.

Need for some Trials that Are Large and Simple and Others that Are Moderate-Sized and more Detailed

The design of any randomized clinical trial should reflect the most efficient means of answering the *primary* question that it addresses. Consequently, clinical trials employing a variety of designs and strategies are needed. For example, trials that are aimed at testing the effect of an agent on ejection fraction or exercise tolerance should employ a design that is very different from studies that aim to assess the effects on mortality or major morbidity.

Key Aspects of Design of Studies with Surrogate Endpoints. Randomized trials which are aimed at studying the effect of drugs on exercise tolerance and ejection fraction usually require only a few hundred patients. One should take into account the reproducibility of the test (measurement and test-retest error within patients), the interpatient variability at baseline and during follow-up, the impact of high mortality rates, nonavailability of follow-up studies due to a variety of factors (death, worsening symptoms, refusal to undergo a second test), and nonadherence to study medications. All randomized patients should be accounted for in the analysis, and the results should be presented with and without making allowances for missing data (e.g., by imputing scores). In a study, outcomes such as ejection fraction and exercise tolerance may be measured on several occasions after randomization. Appropriate care should be taken to define the study question and to collect and integrate the data (e.g., use of slopes of change or averages), to correctly answer the questions. Care should be taken to avoid multiplicity or to correct for multiple comparisons (e.g., by using adjustment techniques such as Bonferroni's inequality, etc.). It is desirable to standardize the methods of measurement if marked heterogeneity in measurement technique between different sites or observers is expected. In addition, biases in the collection and analyses of the measurements should be avoided or minimized by use of placebo controls and/or by blinded analyses of tests. By the very nature of the hypotheses being tested in these trials, specialized tests will be required and the entry criteria have to be more restrictive, for example in a heart failure trial in which exercise tolerance is the endpoint, in addition to the usual types of exclusion whereby patients who have contraindication or clear indications for the intervention are not enrolled, it is usual to exclude patients who cannot or are unwilling to exercise and those in whom exercise tolerance is limited by other factors such as claudication or angina. (Such patients need not be excluded from a trial in which mortality is the key outcome of interest.)

Key Aspects of Trials in Which Mortality or Major Morbidity is the Primary Endpoint. The emphasis in trials in which mortality or major morbidity is the key outcome must be very different in its design and conduct [2]. First, the outcomes of interest are relatively rare (10%–15% mortality per year in CHF compared to one endpoint per person who is alive and compliant at the end of the study in surrogate endpoint trials). Second, at best, mortality can be reduced only to a moderate extent (15%, 20%, or 25% risk reductions). Therefore, *these trials must*

Table 2. Practical guidelines regarding key judgments in designing, conducting, and reporting a trial evaluating the effect of a drug on mortality in patients with left ventricular dysfunction and heart failure

What information does a statistician need?
- What will the event rate be in the control group? Obtain an estimate from a number of different sources. Since most trials exclude certain patients (i.e., contraindications to drug, too sick, other disease, need for the drug), arbitrarily assume that the event rate that will be observed in trial will be lower by at least about 30%–40%. For example, 3-year mortality in patients with an EF <0.35 and heart failure in the Coronary Artery Surgery Study was 45%. In designing the Studies of Left Ventricular Dysfunction, the expected mortality rate was about 30% in the control group.
- What will the noncompliance rate be in those given the active drug? It is typical to assume that between 5% and 10% of patients will stop the study medication every year.
- What proportion of the control patients will be prescribed the study drug? This is highly variable and will depend on the specific agent.
- What difference should one try to detect? This should be 15%, 20%, or at most 25% risk reductions before one factors in noncompliance. Taking noncompliance into account reduces the observed differences.

How many patients is the study likely to need using reasonable assumptions?

Assuming 90% power a two-tailed p value of 0.05 ($Z=1.96$) and a 15% overall "drop-in" and 15% "drop-out," the following table gives an estimate of the numbers of patients required to detect various differences depending upon the event rates:

Percent reduction	Total event rate in the control group		
	21%	25%	27%
15%	8300	7400	6500
20%	4600	4100	3600
25%	2900	2600	2300

How does one recruit a large number of patients?
- Involve many hospitals and physicians.
- Use wide entry criteria that maximize patient eligibility.
- Simplify entry procedures.
- Restrict data collection to the bare minimum.

Remember: It is usually much more difficult to recruit than one expects. Despite good intentions, few trials can recruit than one-fifth to one-half of eligible patients unless the study is extraordinarily simplified.

How does one maximize compliance?
- Exclude patients who are unlikely to comply during screening.
- Use simple and flexible drug regimen and follow-up procedures.
- Try to restart study drug in a noncompliant patient if possible.

How does one avoid biases in:
- Entry of patients? Include all randomized patients in the analysis.
- Endpoint ascertainment? Blind treatment allocation when evaluating outcomes, other than mortality.
- Reporting and analysis? Analyze the data primarily by the rules described in the protocol. Report all other analyses as being secondary.

How does one interpret the results?

Interpret the trial results in the context of other similar trials, effect on related endpoints, and known mechanisms.

be much larger *(about 3000–7000 patients) in order to avoid missing clinically worthwhile and plausible benefits (Table 2)*. Because mortality is an easily assessable endpoint without bias, little effort or standardization is required for endpoint ascertainment. Moreover, apart from some key baseline descriptors and data on postrandomization cotherapy and compliance, few other data are required to interpret the results of the trial (see earlier sections). Therefore, in such studies there is little value in detailed data collection or specialized tests per patient. Instead, simplification in data collection and study procedures make it possible to divert more resources to the most important factor that influences the precision of the trial – uncontrolled and random variations in prognosis and in response to therapy of patients after accounting for all known variables [2]. This can be minimized only by increasing study size so that one can ensure that, on average, patients assigned to the active and control groups are identical.

The collective experiences from cardiovascular trials indicate that among patients who have no clear indication or contraindications to a particular therapy, the effect of a treatment in various subgroups of patients is usually in the same direction (i.e., qualitative interactions are rare) although the size of the effect may vary (i.e., quantitative interactions are common). Acceptance of this principle would encourage the entry of a wider group of patients with the disease into a trial [3]. *The combination of fairly wide entry criteria with simplicity in data collection not only makes a large trial more feasible and cost efficient, but it also makes the study results more applicable to clinical practice than a trial which restricts enrollment to only a few types of patients.* Moreover, if there were compelling reasons to examine the effects of treatment in a few key subsets of patients, having broad entry criteria facilitates this by ensuring the inclusion of large numbers of patients into such categories. Table 2 provides some guidelines regarding key judgments that affect the design of a trial evaluating the effect of a drug on mortality.

Avoidance of Biases in the Conduct, Analysis, and Reporting of Clinical Trials

Randomization avoids systematic biases in the allocation of patients to the active and control (or standard therapy) group. When these studies are sufficiently large (a few hundred patients for surrogate endpoint trials and a few thousand patients for mortality trials), random errors can be minimized, and the sensitivity of the study increases. Further, every attempt should be made to preserve the "contrast" between those allocated to receive the active drug compared to controls by maximizing compliance to study drugs and avoiding large imbalances in the use of other drugs that might have an effect on the outcome of interest.

In addition to the above measures, the results of a randomized study are valid only if biases in endpoint ascertainment can be avoided, all randomized patients are included in the analysis, and the types of analyses follow a prespecified plan with full disclosure of all the results. Two types of biases that have occurred in the analysis and reporting of heart failure trials are described below:

1. In trials of surrogate endpoints, some studies have confined analyses to patients who are alive and taking study drugs. This could lead to biases that affect the original comparability of the two groups. First, patients who die were likely to have been "sicker" at entry than those who are alive. The drug may have a beneficial or adverse effect on survival. Therefore, not accounting for dead patients in the analysis ignores the likelihood that the patients who are alive in the two groups may no longer be comparable with regard to disease severity. Even when the numbers of deaths are similar, there is no guarantee that the types of patients who die in the two groups are similar. For example, if an agent increases mortality in patients with severely limited exercise tolerance, it might spuriously appear that the drug was improving exercise capacity because only fewer "sick" patients remain in the treated group compared to the control group. The converse is also true when a treatment reduces mortality. A truly beneficial treatment may appear to have little value if the survivors in the treated group include high-risk patients who would have otherwise died. There is no ideal way around this problem in trials of heart failure (or other diseases with high mortality). One option would be to present the data with imputed scores (e.g., the worst observed scores for dead patients) and also without imputed scores. If consistent results emerge with both types of analysis, one has greater confidence in the conclusion that the study reaches. Among patients who survive, some may not be on the original drug or may be unable to or refuse to undergo the second test. It is possible that such patients might be more severely ill than the remainder of the patients. In all these cases, excluding such patients from the analysis could potentially create biases. In addition to maximizing compliance to the protocol and obtaining outcome data in as many patients as possible, every patient should be accounted for in the analyses as described above. Of course, if in a trial a high proportion of patients (e.g., over one-third) do not have the follow up tests, the results are likely to be influenced greatly by the manner in which the missing values are handled and the interpretation of the study may become very difficult.

2. In trials in which mortality or major morbidity is the main outcome of interest, it is important to include all randomized patients in the analyses. It is also important that the analysis follow the plan that was set up in advance in the protocol. For example, in the CONSENSUS trial the investigators set out to examine the effect of enalapril on 6-month survival [4]. In their report the investigators correctly placed emphasis on the 6-month results although they reported several other analyses. In another study [5] patients were randomized to a control group, to a group receiving prazosin, or to a group receiving the combination of hydralazine and nitrates. The primary analysis stated in the protocol was to examine the effect in the group of patients on the combined vasodilator regimen versus the control group, for which a p value of 0.05 derived from the log-rank test would indicate statistical significance [6]. Secondary analyses comparing each of the two regimen with the control group were planned. These analyses would use a p value of 0.025 to test for statistical significance. Based upon the data presented in the paper, mortality in the prazosin group was similar to that in the control group, and the group receiving isosorbide-dinitrate plus hydralazine showed a lower mortality ($p=0.093$). Therefore, had an analysis been done in accordance with the protocol, although a lower mortality had been observed in

the vasodilator group, it would not have reached conventional levels of statistical significance. Instead, the report focuses mainly upon the comparison of the hydralazine-isosorbide group with the control group. A number of further analyses, some of which were not prespecified, were carried out. One of these analyses reached the significance level of $p=0.049$ (but still not the prestated level of 0.025). Based upon this, the authors claimed that they had clear evidence of benefit with hydralazine and nitrates. An appropriate analysis would clarify which analyses were based upon prestated hypotheses and methods and separate them from other secondary analysis that the authors wish to emphasize. This would give readers the opportunity to judge the weight of the evidence for themselves. One view would be that an interesting trend has been observed which needs confirmation in other published or future studies.

While trying to adhere to prestated rules may appear pedantic, data-derived analyses performed to emphasize a particular result do not give an appropriate indication of the weight of evidence. Instead, such an analysis smacks of betting on a horse after the race is over. Another variation seen in some studies is the overemphasis on retrospectively identified subgroups where the effect appears to be particularly promising. When a trial shows no difference, or a small difference, if enough subgroups are examined, one is bound to find a few in which treatment appears to be beneficial and the difference can appear to reach some conventional level of statistical significance for which post hoc multiple testing or hypothesis testing has not been taken into account.

Such biases in data analyses and presentation are misleading and should be avoided. Analyses that were considered to be important and were stated in the protocol should always be presented. Additional data-derived analyses might be useful to suggest hypotheses for further studies, to test consistency of the results, or to explore physiologic effects. The results of such analyses should not be considered in the same manner as the original hypotheses that were a part of the study design, unless they are striking and reach extreme levels of statistical significance (Z of 3 or 4).

Limitations in Extrapolating from the Results of Studies on Surrogate Endpoints to Major Clinical Outcomes

When the effects of a therapy on a surrogate endpoint such as ejection fraction, exercise tolerance, or ventricular arrhythmia are evaluated, one hopes that favorable effects on these outcomes will lead to a reduction in morbidity or mortality. However, recent experiences from several studies have demonstrated that improvement in surrogate endpoints does not necessarily correlate with clinical benefit. For example, several studies with different inotropic agents (milrinone, dobutamine, xamoterol or enoximone) have shown improvements in exercise tolerance or left ventricular ejection fraction; however, with each of these agents, a trend towards increased mortality is observed. An overview of the various trials of these agents (Table 3) indicates a twofold excess mortality which is statistically

Table 3. Available data on mortality in randomized trials of inotropic agents other than digitalis in heart failure. (From [1, 7] and personal communication, H. Pouleur)

	Number of deaths/number of patients		Risk ratio	p
	Active	Control		
Amrinone	3/102 (2.9%)	2/104 (1.9%)	1.5	–
Milrinone	27/119 (22.7%)	12/111 (10.8%)	2.1	0.02
Dobutamine	15/49 (30.6%)	8/41 (19.5%)	1.6	–
Xamoterol	32/352 (9.1%)	6/164 (3.7%)	2.5	0.02
Total	77/622 (12.4%)	28/420 (6.7%)	1.9	0.001

The above data should be interpreted cautiously as the data are based on only about 1000 patients followed for a relatively short period. Moreover, one cannot be certain that the results of the trials identified are representative of all trials of these agents that were conducted.

significant [1, 7], (personal communication, H. Pouleur). (The data from this overview should be interpreted cautiously because the various inotropic agents have important differences in their mechanism of action. Moreover, the available data are sparse and could be subject to reporting or publication biases.) At the very least, the data indicate that these agents are unlikely to improve survival.

A second relevant example is the trials of antiarrhythmic agents. In patients admitted within the early hours of infarction, ventricular arrhythmia and fibrillation are common. Intravenous or intramuscular lidocaine (or lignocaine) has been shown to markedly reduce the incidence of ventricular arrhythmia. It has therefore been presumed that lidocaine used routinely would reduce the mortality rate by preventing ventricular fibrillation. In an overview of all the randomized trials on a total of about 10000 patients, there were more deaths among treated patients: 82/4616 (1.8%) deaths among patients allocated to receive lidocaine compared to 55/4539 (1.2%) among controls ($p=0.06$) [8]. In a small trial of postinfarction patients with frequent ventricular ectopic beats following myocardial infarction, flecainide and encainide (two class Ic antiarrhythmic agents) were shown to be extremely effective in suppressing arrhythmia [9]. However, in the larger mortality study (Cardiac Arrhythmia Suppression Trial) [10] the group receiving these agents were shown to experience a 3.6-fold excess arrhythmic death or cardiac arrest compared to controls (4.5% in the encainide/flecainide groups versus 1.2% among control patients; $p<0.001$) [10]. Therefore, these data indicate that arrhythmia suppression by itself does not necessarily confer clinical benefit.

The examples discussed in this section reveal that one should be cautious in extrapolating from small trials on surrogate endpoints to clinical benefit. Trials of surrogate endpoints should be seen as a stepping stone to the design of more definitive and larger trials in which morbidity and mortality are the major outcomes of interest.

Clinical Trials as a Framework for Seeking Information on Prognostic Factors, Clinical Course, and Leads to Mechanism

The primary goal of all randomized clinical trials is to assess the effects of therapy on a specific outcome. When large and long-term trials are conducted, the trial may become the largest systematically and prospectively collected database in that particular condition. These data can be used to test the relative prognositc impact of a number of patient characteristics, describe the clinical course of the disease, estimate the rates of different kinds of complications, and sometimes shed light on pathophysiologic mechanisms. For example, the Studies of left Ventricular Dysfunction (SOLVD), in addition to testing the effects of enalapril on survival in about 6750 patients with left ventricular dysfunction ejection fraction (EF) ≤ 0.35) collects data on the clinical course and on a number of specialized tests. It is expected that the study will provide reliable estimates of the influence of simple parameters such as ejection fraction, New York Heart Association functional classification, disease etiology, comorbidity, and age, etc. on 3-year survival and morbidity (e.g., rate of hospitalization for CHF, other cardiovascular complications such as myocardial infarction, thromboembolism, strokes, and noncardiovascular morbidity such as respiratory infections). Data from a number of substudies are already providing new information on mechanisms. A substudy of 300 patients showed that plasma norepinephrine, atrial natriuretic factor and arginine vasopressin (but not renin) were all elevated in patients with asymptomatic left ventricular dysfunction. Renin was elevated only in patients with overt heart failure who were receiving diuretics. This substudy indicates that neurohumural activation precedes the development of overt heart failure in patients with asymptomatic left ventricular function. This observation raises the potential for instituting appropriate therapy at an earlier stage in the disease.

Despite its many advantages, a clinical trial has several potential disadvantages as a database. Patients entering a trial are highly selected because some of the sickest and most unstable patients, those with contraindications to or those who need the study drug are usually not entered. Therefore, the study population is often truncated, making it sometimes more difficult to show associations or to obtain information about the full spectrum of the disease. This problem may be obviated by the creation of a study registry which records information on a broader group of patients. However, creation of a registry is time consuming and increases study costs. Despite this, a registry is likely to be of value and scientifically informative if created in conjunction with one of the first large trials of a particular condition. Such a database will serve as a resource for a variety of questions that are clinically important and also help in the design of future trials (e.g., event rates, practice styles, definition of a high-risk or target population for a certain type of intervention).

Some Examples of Ongoing Moderate-Sized and Large Trials

Table 4 summarizes the large trials that are currently underway among patients with left ventricular dysfunction. Of these, SOLVD is the largest; it consists of two trials and a patient registry. In both trials patients with an EF ≤0.35 are randomized to receive enalapril, an angiotensin converting enzyme inhibitor, or placebo. The "treatment" trial of SOLVD has randomized 2568 patients who have signs and symptoms of heart failure. The "prevention" trial of SOLVD is expected to randomize approximately 4200 patients without overt heart failure by May 1990. The primary goal of each trial is to assess the effect of enalapril on long-term mortality. In addition, the combined mortality from both trials is considered to be a key and the most important secondary endpoint. Subsidiary aims of the study are to assess the effects of treatment on cardiovascular mortality, deaths due to arrhythmia or progressive heart failure, worsening of heart failure requiring hospitalization, and quality of life. In the prevention trial, onset of heart failure is an additional endpoint. In addition to the main trials, seven structured and detailed substudies are being conducted using subsets of patients. The results of these studies should be available in 1991.

The Study to Avoid Ventricular Enlargement (SAVE) includes patients with an EF ≤0.40 following myocardial infarction. A total of 2200 patients are expected to be randomized to captopril or placebo by January 1990. At the end of 2 years, the effect of treatment on ejection fraction will be evaluated. Results are

Table 4. Some major ongoing or planned trials in patients with left ventricular dysfunction

Vasodilators

- SOLVD (Studies of Left Ventricular Dysfunction) treatment trial ($n=2568$): effect of ACE inhibitors on mortality in CHF patients with EF ≤0.35
- SOLVD prevention trial ($n=4200$): effect of ACE inhibitor on mortality in patients with EF ≤0.35, but no overt CHF
- SAVE (Study to Avoid Ventricular Enlargement) ($n=2200$): effect of ACE inhibitor on the combined endpoint of mortality plus change in EF by 5% among post-MI patients with EF ≤0.40
- V-HeFT-2 (Veterans Heart Failure Trial) ($n=900$): comparison of ACE inhibitors versus hydralazine + nitrates on multiple endpoints among CHF patients (NYHA classes II, III)

Inotropic agents

- PROMISE (Prospective Randomized Milrinone Survival Evaluation) ($n=$ca. 1000): effect of milrinone on mortality among CHF patients (NYHA classes III, IV)
- DIG (Digitalis Investigation Group) ($n=7000$)[a]: effect of digitalis on mortality and CHF hospitalization among CHF patients with EF ≤0.45

Antiarrhythmic agents

- Veterans Administration trial of amiodarone ($n=800$): effect of Amiodarone on mortality in CHF patients (NYHA classes II, III)
- MDC (Metoprolol in Dilated Cardiomyopathy) ($n=400$): effect of metoprolol on mortality in CHF patients

[a] In planning; all other studies are either enrolling patients or have completed recruitment.

expected in the spring of 1992. The data from this trial and those of the SOLVD trials should complement each other.

The Veterans Administration Cooperative Program is conducting two trials – one comparing enalapril with the combination of hydralazine and isosorbide on exercise tolerance, ejection fraction, and quality of life in 900 NYHA class II and III patients (V-HeFT-2) and the second comparing the effects of amiodarone with placebo in patients with heart failure in preventing mortality and arrhythmic death. The first study is expected to report in 1992; the latter study is recruiting patients.

PROMISE (Prospective Randomized Milrinone Survival Evaluation) is a study of about 1000 patients with NYHA class III and IV heart failure evaluating the role of milrinone on survival among patients already on an ACE inhibitor. This study had recruited 450 patients by October 1989. Results are expected by early 1991.

The Metoprolol in Dilated Cardiomyopathy Study is evaluating whether metoprolol compared to placebo improves survival among patients with idiopathic dilated cardiomyopathy. This trial has recruited about 200 out of an expected total of 400 patients. Results are expected in 1991 ore 1992. A few groups have been planning large studies with beta-blockers and magnesium, but these studies are unlikely to start until the middle of 1990.

There is an urgent need to evaluate the role of digoxin on survival and morbidity in patients with heart failure and sinus rhythm. A large study is currently being developed by the National Heart, Lung and Blood Institute in conjunction with the Veterans Administration Cooperative Studies Program and Burroughs-Wellcome to evaluate this question.

Conclusions and Recommendations

Until recently there have been few large randomized trials in patients with left ventricular dysfunction and heart failure. Such studies are essential in order to obtain reliable estimates of the effects of various treatments on mortality or morbidity. Extrapolation from the effects of drugs on surrogate endpoints to clinically important outcomes is not trustworthy because improvements in exercise capacity, ejection fraction, or arrhythmias do not necessarily lead to reductions in mortality or morbidity. Because even the most promising agents are likely to have only a moderate benefit (e.g., 15%–20% risk reduction) on long-term (i.e., several years) mortality or morbidity, large trials involving several thousands of patients followed for a few years are required. Development of collaborative structures by which sufficient numbers of patients can be entered quickly and at a reasonable cost into each study is an important challenge that faces researchers and clinicians in this field.

References

1. Furberg CD, Yusuf S (1988) Effect of drug therapy on survival in chronic congestive heart failure. Am J Cardiol 62:42A–45A
2. Yusuf S, Collins R, Peto R (1984) Why do we need some large, simple randomized trials? Stat Med 3:409–420
3. Yusuf S, Held P, Teo KK, Toretsky ER (1990) Selection of patients for randomized controlled trials: implications of wide or narrow eligibility criteria. Stat Med 9:73–86
4. CONSENSUS Trial Study Group (1987) Effects of enalapril on mortality in severe congestive heart failure. N Engl J Med 316:1429–1435
5. Cohn JN, Archibald DG, Ziesche S et al. (1986) Effect of vasodilator therapy on mortality in chronic congestive heart failure: results of a Veterans Administration Cooperative Study. N Engl J Med 314:1547–1552
6. Protocol for VA Cooperative Study no 153. Vasodilator used in chronic congestive heart failure. February 1982:1–59
7. DiBianco R, Shabetai R, Kostuk W, Moran J, Schlant RC, Wright R for the Milrinone Multicenter Trial (1989) A comparison of oral milrinone, digoxin and their combination in the treatment of patients with chronic heart failure. N Engl J Med 320:677–683
8. MacMahon S, Collins R, Peto R, Koster RW, Yusuf S (1988) Effects of prophylactic lidocaine in suspected acute myocardial infarction. An overview of results from the randomized controlled trials. JAMA 260:1910–1916
9. Cardiac Arrhythmia Pilot Study (CAPS) Investigators (1988) Effects of encainide, flecainide, imipramine and moricizine on ventricular arrhythmias during the year after acute myocardial infarction: the CAPS. Am J Cardiol 61:501–509
10. Cardiac Arrhythmia Suppression Trial (CAST) Investigators (1989) Preliminary report: effect of encainide and flecainide on mortality in a randomized trial of arrhythmia suppression after myocardial infarction. N Engl J Med 321:406–412

Prognostic Significance of Asymptomatic Ventricular Arrhythmias in Heart Failure: Potential for Mortality Reduction by Pharmacologic Control*

B. N. SINGH, M. P. SCHOENBAUM, M. ANTIMISIARIS, and C. TAKANAKA

Introduction

That patients surviving acute myocardial infarction incur an increased incidence of sudden death especially in the first 6 months to 1 year [1, 2] is well known. The highest risk is in patients with markedly reduced ejection fraction particularly in association with complex ventricular ectopy [3, 4]. Although not entirely certain, it appears that ventricular arrhythmias in this setting are associated with an enhanced mortality from sudden death independently of left ventricular dysfunction [3]. In recent years attention has turned towards the prognostic significance of asymptomatic ventricular arrhythmias in patients with overt cardiac failure [5, 6] especially in those with NYHA classes III and IV of functional disability. As in the case of survivors of acute infarction, they too appear to be markers of increased mortality from sudden death [6, 7–14]. The issue has become of major importance because the mortality rate for patients with congestive heart failure is extremely high, being about 50% in the 1st year following referral for treatment of patients with class III or IV functional disability [3]. About 40% of such deaths are sudden [15, 17].

Such sudden deaths are not influenced by vasodilator therapy, which does however exert a beneficial effect on deaths related to heart failure [18, 20]. The implication is that sudden deaths in this setting are arrhythmic in nature, and that vasodilators are devoid of intrinsic antiarrhythmic properties. The purpose of this chapter is to discuss briefly the prognostic significance and the potential pharmacologic approaches to mortality reduction by the control of asymptomatic ventricular arrhythmias in patients with congestive heart failure.

Prevalence and Prognostic Significance

Many studies have reported a high incidence of potentially lethal ventricular arrhythmias – ventricular couplets, multiform complexes, and nonsustained ventricular tachycardia – in patients with dilated cardiomyopathy and in those with

---

* Supported by the Medical Research Service of the Veterans Administration and the American Heart Association of the Greater Los Angeles Affiliate.

heart failure due to ischemic heart disease [6–14, 21–23]. The incidence of complex ventricular ectopy has ranged between 12% and 95% in various reports [15]; the incidence of nonsustained ventricular tachycardia has been similar [15]. In contrast, the incidence of nonsustained ventricular tachycardia is about 10% 2 weeks after an acute infarction. In nearly every study, in patients with nonsustained ventricular tachycardia there was a higher total or sudden death rate compared to those who did not have the arrhythmia. Interestingly, patients having ventricular tachycardia ran three times the risk of dying as those without the tachycardia. Furthermore, during follow-up, patients with ventricular tachycardia also had a higher mortality in every study. These data suggested that the effect on mortality was independent of the clinical severity of heart failure. This was also suggested by the preliminary data of the Veterans Administration Cooperative Study of the effect of vasodilator therapy on mortality in congestive cardiac failure [24]. The question has therefore arisen whether the suppression of such arrhythmias documented on Holter recordings may prolong survival over and above that induced by vasodilator therapy in patients with congestive cardiac failure.

Mechanisms of Sudden Death in Heart Failure

Implicit in the belief that it might be possible to alter the course of arrhythmic deaths in heart failure is that the mechanism of such deaths is known. There is however controversy regarding the precise nature of the preterminal events in the development of the sudden death syndrome in individual patients. From the analysis of Holter recordings in patients dying suddenly while wearing Holter monitors, a number of features have been identified [25]. There is evidence that although the largest number of patients dying suddenly have coronary artery disease, the initiating event is not triggered by readily identifiable episodes of myocardial ischemia [25]. Ventricular tachycardia episodes are triggered by ventricular ectopic beats. Most cases of sudden death which have occurred while the patient was wearing the Holter device have shown that the initial arrhythmia is ventricular tachycardia which deteriorates promptly into ventricular fibrillation (Fig. 1) as a result of acceleration of the tachycardia [13, 25]. It must nevertheless be emphasized that while an episode of myocardial ischemia does not appear to be the immediate cause of the ventricular tachycardia, it may provide the basis for its degeneration into fibrillation especially in the setting of augmented adrenergic activity. These considerations are based on observations in patients incurring out-of-hospital sudden death while wearing Holter monitoring. Although such patients almost invariably have reduced ventricular ejection fractions, rarely are they in frank heart failure. Thus, it is possible that the sequence of events mediating sudden death in patients with frank heart failure may differ. Indeed, in-hospital monitoring of heart failure patients awaiting cardiac transplantation has indicated that in many patients profound bradycardia and asystole rather than ventricular tachycardia or fibrillation constitutes the terminal event (Fig. 2). For example, Luu et al. [26] recently reported an unexpectedly high incidence of

Heart Failure, Arrhythmias and Prognosis

Fig. 1. The sequence of electrocardiographic abnormalities during the development of sudden death in a patient with dilated cardiomyopathy. The patient was wearing a Holter monitor at the time that he developed cardiac arrest. Note that the onset of the ventricular tachycardia was initiated by a premature ventricular tachycardia (*VT*); the first episode was nonsustained. The second episode deteriorated into ventricular fibrillation by the shortening of the cycle length of the VT. (From [13])

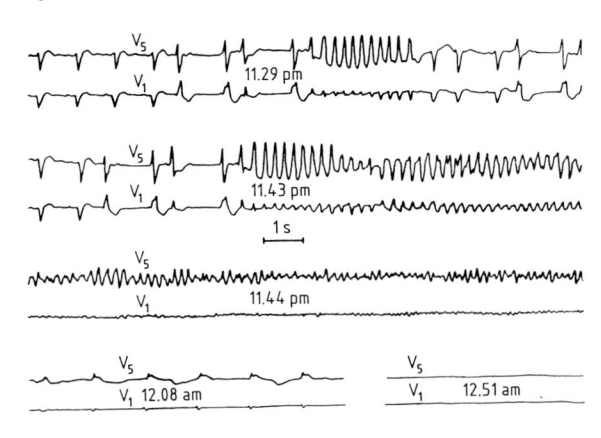

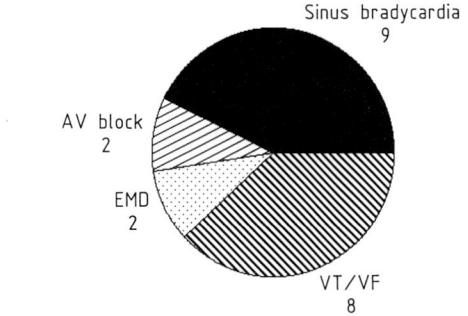

Fig. 2. Initial rhythm at 21 cardiac arrests in patients with advanced heart failure being monitored in hospital while awaiting cardiac transplantation. (From [26])

bradycardia and asystole in patients with heart failure (mean left ventricular ejection fraction 18%) awaiting cardiac transplantation. Over a 4-year period there were 20 deaths from a population of 216 (9%). In only 38% was the terminal event associated with ventricular tachycardia deteriorating into ventricular tachycardia. In 62% the rhythm at the time of arrest was severe bradycardia or electromechanical dissociation. Clearly, if these data can be confirmed with a larger series, it may have a significant bearing on the issue of attempts at mortality reduction by the use of antiarrhythmic drugs. The use of automatic implantable cardioverter-defibrillators with pacemaking capability might be more appropriate if such patients prone to bradycardic deaths can be identified prospectively.

Pharmacologic Approaches and Impact on Survival

A clear distinction should be made between the treatment of sustained ventricular arrhythmias associated with symptoms and those that are nonsustained and asymptomatic. In the former, treatment is for the relief of symptoms with the expectation of prolonging survival. The role of electrophysiologic testing in the design of therapy is widely used, although controversies remain. In the latter (the group under discussion here), the sole objective of therapy is enhanced survival presumably by the suppression of spontaneously occurring ventricular arrhythmias. The role of electrophysiologic testing in this subset of patients is questionable. It is known that angiotensin-converting enzyme inhibitors do increase serum potassium levels, reduce the augmented plasma catecholamine levels, and produce a concomitant decrease in PVCs and runs of nonsustained ventricular tachycardia [27]. The fact that this does not lead to a reduction in the incidence of sudden death (versus cardiac and total deaths which are reduced) may suggest that a reduction in PVCs is unlikely to result in a fall in the rate of sudden deaths in this setting. Alternatively, vasodilators may not exert a primary antifibrillatory action in the setting of cardiac disease.

It is widely recognized that beta-blockers, at least those which exert a heart rate lowering effect under resting conditions, reduce the incidence of sudden death in the survivors of acute myocardial infarction [28]. Whether this class of agents might exert a similar effect in heart failure remains uncertain. Three small trials (two using metoprolol and one acebutalol) have demonstrated that very small doses of beta-blockers appear to produce symptomatic improvement in a subset of patients with dilated cardiomyopathy [29–31]. The limited mortality data from these trials when pooled indicated a trend in favor of treatment, but no definitive conclusions could be reached [32]. A larger trial, the Multi-center Metoprolol in Dilated Cardiomyopathy Study, is currently ongoing with the aim of enrolling 320 patients to be randomized into metoprolol and placebo arms over a 2-year period (J. L. Anderson 1989, personal communication).

Arrhythmia Suppression and Mortality in Heart Failure

No controlled trials have been done to test the hypothesis that the suppression of such arrhythmias in these patients will reduce the incidence of sudden death. The results of uncontrolled albeit small studies have yielded conflicting data.

Parmley and Chatterjee [33] analyzed the incidence of sudden deaths in a subgroup of patients with heart failure and complex ventricular ectopic beats. The patients were treated with quinidine or procainamide ($n=26$) or with amiodarone ($n=13$). The treated group had a cumulative survival rate of 90%–95% at 6 months compared with approximately 65% in patients not receiving antiarrhythmic therapy. The difference was significant ($p<0.05$). In another study reported by Dargie et al. [34], the presence of ventricular ectopic activity in patients with heart failure was a strong predictor for subsequent cardiac death. Furthermore, a comparison of groups of such patients on treatment with amiodarone with those not treated with antiarrhythmic agents showed a significant difference in favor of amiodarone which not only reduced ventricular ectopy but also prolonged survival. In contrast, Chakko and Georghiade [12] followed 43 patients with chronic heart failure due to dilated cardiomyopathy; 88% of the patients had complex ventricular ectopic activity with 51% having nonsustained asymptomatic ventricular tachycardia. Twenty-three of the patients received long-term antiarrhythmic therapy with procainamide or quinidine, and 20 were not treated. The two groups were comparable. At a mean follow-up period of 16 months, there were 16 deaths, 62% sudden. There was no significant difference between the numbers of such deaths in the treated and untreated groups.

It must be emphasized that these studies are severely limited by the numbers of patients, lack of adequate controls, and standardization of therapy. They merely indicate that the data support the idea of a stringently controlled study with adequate sample size and statistical power that should be undertaken to test the hypothesis that antiarrhythmic therapy reduces the mortality from sudden death in patients with cardiac failure, and that such an effect is linked to a suppression of complex ventricular ectopic activity. However, there is no unanimity of opinion regarding the choice of antiarrhythmic agents that might be used as electropharmacologic probes to address these fundamental questions. Nonetheless, there are numerous considerations which bear on the issue, not the least being the preliminary data from the Cardiac Arrhythmia Suppression Trial (CAST) in the United States in patients surviving acute myocardial infarction.

Lessons from the Cardiac Arrhythmia Suppression Trial: To Depress Conduction or to Prolong Refractoriness?

Although the preliminary results of CAST are from a different subset of patients with asymptomatic ventricular arrhythmias, they have an important bearing on the treatment of similar arrhythmias in patients with cardiac failure. The aim of CAST was to test the PVC hypothesis, i.e., the suppression of premature ventricular contractions by antiarrhythmic agents in the survivors of acute infarction reduces the incidence of sudden cardiac death. The test drugs were flecainide, encainide, ethmozine, and placebo.

Flecainide and encainide were selected for the trial because these drugs produce a predictable suppression of PVCs: in about 80% of patients there is over 75% suppression of total PVCs, over 90% suppression of ventricular couplets, and close to 100% suppression of ventricular tachycardia beats. Ethmozine was selected because of its favorable side effects profile and its modest PVC suppressant action. Thus, in the asymptomatic patient with complex PVCs with increased risk for sudden arrhythmic deaths, encainide and similar drugs provided the basis for CAST under the aegis of the National Heart Lung and Blood Institute's Clinical Trials Branch in Bethesda, Maryland. In the event, after 2 years into the study, it appeared that rather than reducing the incidence of death in the group with encainide or flecainide, there was an *increase* in mortality when compared to the effects of placebo. The preliminary results of the trial involving 1500 patients at 23 centers in the United States, Canada, and Sweden revealed that of the 730 patients assigned to encainide or flecainide and treated an average of 10 months, 56 had died or suffered cardiac arrest, while among the 725 given a placebo 23 had died or suffered cardiac arrest. It also appeared that the effects of ethmozine (a less powerful PVC suppressant and a less powerful depressant of conduction) were not deleterious. The difference in the case of encainide and flecainide is disturbing and cannot be ignored. They have been withdrawn from the trial, which is continuing. These results leave the clinician in considerable confusion regarding the role of PVC suppression by agents which selectively and markedly delay conduction as a modality of therapy of asymptomatic PVCs in the expectation of reducing sudden deaths in the survivors of acute infarction.

What are the implications of the results of CAST for design of studies to determine whether antiarrhythmic therapy might have an impact on sudden death in patients with cardiac failure? Several issues should be considered. First, it is clear that the degree of slowing of conduction induced by flecainide and encainide in patients with ventricular arrhythmias is perhaps excessive; while these drugs clearly have a powerful suppressant effect on reducing the trigger mechanisms for the initiation of the sustained tachyarrhythmia, they appear to make the substrate more prone to develop focal reexcitation. It might be speculated that these drugs have little effect on the genesis of PVCs; it is likely they merely prevent their propagation so that they are not "seen" on the surface electrocardiogram. The excessive slowing of conduction induced by class Ic agents in concert with their differential effects on the action potential duration in Purkinje's fibers and the ventricular muscle – shortening in the former and lengthening it in the latter [35, 36] – might provide the background to their proarrhythmic actions. This overall action results in marked heterogeneity in excitability and refractoriness in the myocardium which is likely to be particularly significant in the context of disease. The CAST data indicate an urgent need to determine the mechanisms underlying the proarrhythmic actions of class I agents in general and to define the extent of slowing of conduction that might be beneficial and the limit at which it is likely to become deleterious.

Second, the data raise the issue, suspected for sometime, that the reduction of PVCs (it being doubtful whether it is indeed possible to eliminate every PVC that is generated in the heart), may not lead directly to a reduction in sudden death. The CAST results support this premise, at least with respect to the drugs that have a marked propensity to slow conduction. On the other hand, the possibility is not excluded that reduction or elimination in repetitive beats by agents which have a different electrophysiologic profile with no effect on conduction (e.g., beta-blockers) or those with modest depressant effect on conduction (e.g., amiodarone) might be effective in altering mortality in patients with potentially life-threatening ventricular arrhythmias. It remains to be determined as to how much slowing of conduction in this setting is beneficial, and at what level of change in conduction in any subset of patients it begins to be deleterious. Finally, the results with encainide and flecainide in CAST do provide a further impetus for considering agents which modify the other "end" of the action potential (potassium-channel blockers) in the control of malignant ventricular arrhythmias [36–42]. The focus here is on homogenously increasing refractoriness by prolonging the action potential duration in the substrate but without the tendency for membrane oscillation leading to torsades de pointes [13]. Such an approach might lead to the development of effective pharmacologic regimens for altering mortality from ventricular arrhythmias by their antifibrillatory properties without a *major* effect on conduction in the heart [41].

Characteristics of a Desirable Antiarrhythmic Agent for Mortality Reduction in Cardiac Failure

In the design of an anti-arrhythmic regimen for mortality reduction in patients with heart failure and potentially lethal ventricular arrhythmias two main factors merit considerations: the pathophysiologic mechanisms of heart failure having a bearing on the genesis of arrhythmias and the electrophysiologic and pharmacodynamic properties of antiarrhythmic compounds. Electrolyte disturbances and the derangements of the autonomic nervous system are clearly important. The electrolyte abnormalities may result not only from persistent diuretic therapy but also as a result of the stimulation of the renin-angiotensin system [34, 43]. It has long been known that the sympathetic nervous system is activated in heart failure in proportion to the severity of cardiac failure [34, 43], there being a relationship between plasma norepinephrine levels and survival in these patients. The choice of an antiarrhythmic compound in the setting of heart failure must clearly allow for the fact that it is nearly impossible to restore complete normality of homeostasis with respect to electrolytes and plasma norepinephrine levels. Electrolyte disturbances, especially hypokalemia and hypomagnesemia, may not only reduce the efficacy of certain antiarrhythmic agents (especially class I agents) but may aggravate the tendency for proarrhythmic effects both for class I (ventricular tachycardia and fibrillation) and class III (torsades de pointes) agents. The arrhythmogenic effects of elevated plasma catecholamines is well known; it is also known that attenuation of the effects of adrenergic stimulation by whatever means has beneficial effects in cardiac arrhythmias. Thus, in the choice of an agent it might be desirable to select one that does have the additional property of inhibiting adrenergic drive while eliminating either the trigger mechanisms for ventricular arrhythmias or conferring on the myocardium an antifibrillatory propensity by selectively prolonging refractoriness.

It is almost trite to emphasize that the side effects profile of the agent to be used in cardiac failure needs to acceptable. On the other hand, since the arrhythmia mortality is inordinately high in this group of patients, the spectrum and severity of side effects that might be acceptable for an effective antiarrhythmic agent in this setting are clearly different from those in subsets of patients with a lower potential for sudden cardiac death. It is nevertheless clear that antiarrhythmic agents for patients with heart failure should not have the proclivity to depress ventricular function and exacerbate cardiac failure. For this reason it is unlikely that class I agents as an electrophysiologic class and *full* doses of beta-blockers are likely to become the mainstay of therapy for arrhythmias in patients with severe heart failure. In contrast, class III agents (not necessarily so-called "pure" class III agents) as a group appear to exert a very much lower potential to depress hemodynamic function or to aggravate existing cardiac failure. They also appear to have more clearly definable, predictable, and, in many cases, perhaps more manageable proarrhythmic effects than those exhibited by potent class I agents.

Class III Antiarrhythmic Drugs and Mortality Reduction from Sudden Death in Heart Failure: Significance of Amiodarone Action

The available clinical and experimental electropharmacologic data indicate the potential importance of agents that appear to act by prolonging effective refractory period by an uniform lengthening of cardiac repolarization. The list of such agents is growing. The expanding appeal of these agents stems from a number of factors. First, because these agents as a class augment myocardial contractility [35, 39], they are clearly desirable from the standpoint that the greatest number of patients at the highest risk for sudden arrhythmic deaths have reduced ventricular function. Second, this is also the subset of patients with the highest potential for developing proarrhythmic actions in the case of class I agents in general. The proarrhythmic effects of class III agents are confined essentially to torsades de pointes, an arrhythmia that appears to be a specific proarrhythmic consequence of prolonged cardiac repolarization. It is not always fatal. Third, the fundamental action of class III drugs is unlikely to be linked solely or even in a major way to the suppression of PVCs [41, 42]. The results of CAST [44] have suggested that such an approach based on a defined extent of PVC suppression is now in difficulty. It is possible and indeed likely that the potentially salutary antifibrillatory effects of class III compounds may occur entirely independently of the suppression of PVCs. The available data indicate that the so-called "pure" class III agents are weak PVC suppressants [41]. Their effects on PVCs should not be compared with those of other class III agents such as sotalol and amiodarone which have additional properties having an influence on PVCs independently of their propensity to prolong cardiac repolarization and refractoriness. This is particularly so in the case of amiodarone which has a powerful suppressant effect on PVCs, a marked lengthening effect on refractoriness, a bradycardic action, and an antiischemic potential almost comparable to that of beta-blockers.

Preliminary data on the effects of amiodarone in heart failure [34], in hypertrophic cardiomyopathy [45], in survivors of acute myocardial infarction [46], and particularly in patients with recalcitrant ventricular tachycardia and fibrillation [40, 47] indicate its potential to reduce the rate of sudden deaths in patients with heart failure. A few details of these studies merit emphasis. Although the numbers of patients studied were small, the data reported by Dargie et al. [34] indicated that those in heart failure having frequent and complex PVCs had a lower rate of survival than those in whom the PVCs were fewer. Furthermore, they noted that the survival was significantly improved by the administration of chronic amiodarone therapy. These uncontrolled data are in line with those in hypertrophic cardiomyopathy reported by McKenna et al. [45]. In this study the authors compared the effects of amiodarone on survival in patients with hypertrophic cardiomyopathy and asymptomatic nonsustained ventricular tachycardia with historical controls. The control series comprised 86 patients, of whom 24 were found to have ventricular tachycardia on Holter monitoring; they were given conventional antiarrhythmic drugs. During a 3-year follow up seven died. Of these, five had continued to have ventricular tachycardia, and two had none. In another series of 81 patients, ventricular tachycardia was found in 21 patients who subsequently received amiodarone (150–400 mg/day; median dose 300 mg/day) which suppressed ventricular tachycardia in all 21 patients. There were two deaths, but neither patient was taking amiodarone at the time of sudden death. Thus, the data indicated that amiodarone even in this small patient population exerted what appeared to be a marked effect on the incidence of sudden death while suppressing runs of asymptomatic ventricular tachycardia.

In relation to the results of CAST [44], the very recent preliminary data of Burkart et al. [46] are clearly of major importance. They screened 1210 consecutive patients with myocardial infarction and found 330 (27%) who had persistent asymptomatic ventricular arrhythmias (Lown class equal to or greater than III) about the time of discharge from hospital. Of these, 312 patients were randomized to three treatment arms: no treatment ($n=114$), conventional therapy with class I antiarrhythmic therapy ($n=100$) in a regimen to provide a defined degree of arrhythmia suppression, and amiodarone (200–400 mg/day after a loading dose of 1000 mg/day for 5 days). There were 98 patients in this group. At the end of 12 months of follow-up, there were 15 deaths in the no-treatment group, 12 in the group given conventional class I agents, and 5 in the group given amiodarone. Based on the intention-to-treat principle, the probability for survival for the patients given amiodarone was significantly improved when compared to the no-treatment group ($p<0.01$). This held true for total as well as for sudden deaths. It was of interest that the mortality reduction for sudden death was more pronounced than for total deaths, suggesting that the salutary effect of amiodarone might be related primarily to its antiarrhythmic properties. Although these data are preliminary and only partially controlled, they stand in sharp contrast to those reported in the CAST study in which powerful PVC suppressants were used.

These findings, of course, require confirmation although they are in line with the findings in other subsets of patients and with those in experimental animals [48, 49]. It is generally agreed that the severest test of an antiarrhythmic agent is its efficacy in the survivors of out-of-hospital sudden death. We have followed 72 such patients for a period of 96 months. They were treated with amiodarone when other antiarrhythmic agents had not been effective. Although there was no concurrent controls, there was a lower attrition rate from sudden death of 5% per year, again indicating the possibility of a major beneficial effect on the incidence of sudden death.

Finally, it should be emphasized that the proarrhythmic effect of the drug is low compared to either class I agents or to other class III agents, most of which induce at least a 5% incidence of torsades de pointes [42]. In the case of amiodarone, it appears to be less than 2%, occurring essentially in the setting of marked hypokalemia or when administered in association with drugs that further prolong cardiac repolarization or depress conduction. It is truly remarkable that despite the fact that the drug may prolong the QT interval to over 600 ms and produce a profound degree of tachycardia, the incidence of torsade de pointes remains low [41]. The reason for this is not clear at present, but preliminary data recently reported by Takanaka and Singh [46] have suggested that it may in part be related to the calcium antagonistic effects of amiodarone inhibiting the

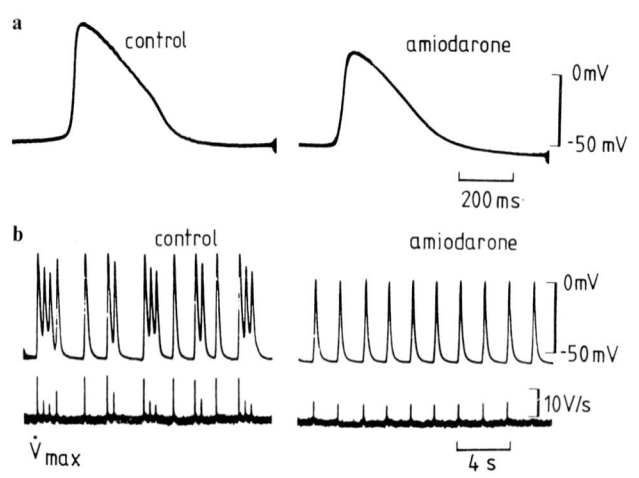

Fig. 3. a *Control*, an action potential due to abnormal automaticity recorded in control solution. *Amiodarone*, an action potential recorded 90 min after the initiation of amiodarone at 5.0×10^{-5} M. There was no significant change in the action potential duration, although the amplitude of the action potential decreased considerably.
b *Control*, action potentials and V_{max} in the control solution recorded from a preparation belonging to the "irregular group." *Amiodarone*, 90 min after the initiation of amiodarone at 5.0×10^{-5} M. Amiodarone totally precluded the development of additional depolarizations. (From [50])

propensity for the development of early afterdepolarizations responsible for torsades (see Fig. 3).

The overall electrophysiologic properties of amiodarone, despite its complex side effects profile, have therefore formed the basis for considering it the best antiarrhythmic agent for determining the effects of therapy on the incidence of sudden death in patients with arrhythmias complicating cardiac failure. Such a blinded placebo-controlled study has recently been initiated under aegis of the Veterans Administration Cooperative Study Section. The study design is entirely different from CAST insofar as the entry requirement is not linked to a defined degree of PVC suppression. However, all patients entering the study will require the presence of a certain minimum number of PVCs under baseline conditions. Serial Holter recordings will be done, but the results of the Holter analysis will not influence decision making with respect to the conduct of the study once the patient has been enrolled into the trial. The major end points of the trial will be sudden death and total cardiac deaths. The data obtained will, however, allow a retrospective analysis of the potential relationship between arrhythmia suppression and the effects on mortality. The results will clearly be of importance in establishing whether antifibrillatory and antiarrhythmic therapy exert an influence on sudden arrhythmic deaths in patients with congestive cardiac failure.

Acknowledgement. I am much indebted to Lawrence Kimble for help with the preparation of this chapter.

References

1. Ruberman W, Weinblatt E, Goldberg J (1977) Ventricular premature beats and mortality after acute myocardial infarction. N Engl J Med 293:750–755
2. Moss AJ, Davis HT, DeCamilla J (1977) Ventricular ectopic beats and their relation to sudden and non-sudden death after myocardial infarction. Circulation 60:998–1004
3. Bigger JT Jr, Fleiss JL, Kleiger R, Miller JP, Rolnitzky LM (1984) The Multicenter Post-Infarction Group: the relationship between ventricular arrhythmias, left ventricular dysfunction and mortality in the two years after myocardial infarction. Circulation 69:250
4. Mukharji J, Rude RE, Poole WK, Gustafson N, Thomas LJ Jr, Strauss HW, Jaffe AS, Muller JE, Roberts R, Raabe DS Jr, Croft CH, Passamani E, Braunwald E, Willerson JT, and the MILIS Study Group (1984) Risk factors for sudden death after acute myocardial infarction: two year follow-up. Am J Cardiol 54:31–37
5. McKenna WJ, England D, Doi YL, Deanfield JE, Oakley CM, Goodwin JF (1981) Arrhythmia in hypertrophy cardiomyopathy. Influence on prognosis. Br Heart J 46:168–172
6. Maskin CS, Siskind SJ, LeJemptel TH (1984) High prevalence of nonsustained ventricular tachycardia in severe congestive heart failure. Am Heart J 107:896–902
7. Wilson JR, Schwartz, Sutton MS-J, Ferrao N, Horowaitz LN, Reichek N, Josephson ME (1983) Prognosis in severe heart failure: relationship to hemodynamic measurements and ventricular ectopic activity. J Am Coll Cardiol 2:403
8. Von Olshausen K, Schafer A, Mehmel HC, Schwartz F, Senges J, Kubler W (1984) Ventricular arrhythmias in idiopathic dilated cardiomyopathy. Br Heart J 51:195
9. Franciosa JA, Wilen M, Ziesche SM, Cohn JN (1983) Survival in men with severe chronic left ventricular failure due to either coronary heart disease or idiopathic dilated cardiomyopathy. Am J Cardiol 51:831
10. Huang SK, Messer JV, Denes P (1983) Significance of ventricular tachycardia in idiopathic dilated cardiomyopathy: observations in 35 patients. Am J Cardiol 51:507
11. Francis GS (1983) Development of arrhythmias in the patient with congestive heart failure: pathophysiology, prevalence and prognosis. Am J Cardiol 51:507
12. Chakko CS, Gheorghiade M (1985) Ventricular arrhythmias in severe heart failure: incidence, significance, and effectiveness of antiarrhythmic therapy. Am Heart J 109:497
13. Meinertz T, Hofman T, Kasper W, Treese N, Bechtold H, Stienen U, Pop T, Leitner E-RV, Andersen D, Meyer J (1984) Significance of ventricular arrhythmias in idiopathic dilated cardiomyopathy. Am J Cardiol 53:902
14. Holmes J, Kubo SH, Cody RJ, Kligfield P (1985) Arrhythmias in ischemic and non-ischemic dilated cardiomyopathy: prediction of mortality by ambulatory electrocardiography. Am J Cardiol 55:146
15. Bigger JT (1987) Why some patients with congestive heart failure die: arrhythmias and sudden cardiac death. Circulation 75 [Suppl IV]:28–35
16. Unverferth DV, Magorein RD, Moeschberger ML, Baker PB, Fetters JK, Leier CV (1984) Factors influencing the one-year mortality of dilated cardiomyopathy. Am J Cardiol 54:147
17. Bigger JT Jr, Weld RM, Rolnitzky LM (1981) The prevalence and significance of ventricular tachycardia detected by ambulatory ECG recording in the hospital phase of acute myocardial infarction. Am J Cardiol 48:815
18. Cohn JN, Archibald DF, Ziesche S, Franciosa JA, Harston WE, Tristani FE, Dunkman WB, Jacobs W, Francis GS, Flohr KH, Goldman S, Cobb FR, Shah PM, Saunders R, Fletcher RD, Loeb HS, Hughes VC, Baker B (1986) Effect of vasodilator therapy on mortality in chronic congestive heart failure. Results of a Veterans Administration Cooperative Study. N Engl J Med 314:1547
19. CONSENSUS Trial Study Group (1987) Effects of enalapril on mortality in severe congestive heart failure: result of the Cooperative North Scandinavian Enalapril Survival Study (CONSENSUS). N Engl J Med 316:1429–1435
20. Captopril Multicenter Research Group I (1986) A cooperative multicenter study of captopril in congestive heart failure: hemodynamic effects and long-term response. Am Heart J 110:439–447
21. Sakurari T, Kawai C (1983) Sudden death in idiopathic cardiomyopathy. Jpn Circ J 47:581

22. Francis GS (1986) Development of arrhythmias in the patient with congestive heart failure: pathophysiology, prevalence and prognosis. Am J Cardiol 57:3B–7B
23. Buxton AE, Marchlinski FE, Waxman HL, Flores C, Cassidy DM, Josephson ME (1984) Prognostic factors in nonsustained ventricular tachycardia. Am J Cardiol 53:1275
24. Fletcher RD, Archibald D, Orndorff J, Cohn J (1986) Dysrhythmias on short-term Holter as an independent predictor of mortality in congestive heart failure. J Am Coll Cardiol 7:143A (abstr)
25. Bayes de Luna A, Coumel P, Leclerq JF (1987) Ambulatory sudden cardiac death: mechanisms of production of fatal arrhythmia on the basis of data from 157 cases. Am Heart J 117:151–159
26. Luu M, Stevenson WG, Stevenson LW, Baron K, Warden J (1989) Diverse mechanisms of unexpected cardiac arrests in advanced heart failure. Circulation 80:1675–1680
27. Cleland JGF, Dargie HJ, Hodsman GP (1984) Captorpril in heart failure: a double-blind controlled study. Br Heart J 52:530–536
28. Kjekshus J (1987) Heart rate reduction – a mechanism of benefit? Eur Heart J 8 [Suppl 1]:115–122
29. Anderson JL, Lutz JR, Gilbert EM, Sorenson SG, Yanowitz FG, Menlove RL, Bartholomew M (1985) A randomized trial of low-dose beta-blockade therapy for idiopathic dilated cardiomyopathy. Am J Cardiol 55:471–475
30. Currie PJ, Kelly MJ, McKenzie A, Harper RW, Lim YL, Federman J, Anderson ST, Pitt A (1984) Oral beta-adrenergic blockade with metoprolol in chronic severe dilated cardiomyopathy. J Am Coll Cardiol 3:203–209
31. Engelmeier RS, O'Connell JB, Walsh R, Rad N, Scanlon PJ, Gunnar RM (1985) Improvement in symptoms and exercise tolerance by metoprolol in patients with dilated cardiomyopathy: a double-blind, randomized, placebo-controlled trial. Circulation 72:536–546
32. Furberg CD, Yusuf S (1988) Effect of drug therapy on survival in chronic congestive heart failure. Am J Cardiol 62:41A–45A
33. Parmley WW, Chatterjee K (1988) Congestive heart failure and arrhythmias: an overview. Am J Cardiol 57:34B–37B
34. Dargie HJ, Cleland JGF, Leckie BJ, Inglis CG, East BW, Ford I (1987) Relation of arrhythmias and electrolyte abnormalities to survival in patients with severe congestive heart failure. Circulation 75 [Suppl 4]:98–107
35. Singh BN, Courtney K (1990) On the classification of anti-arrhythmic mechanisms: experimental and clinical correlations. In: Zipes DP, Jaliffe J (eds) Cardiac electrophysiology: from the cell to the bedside. Saunders, Philadelphia
36. Singh BN (1987) Effects of anti-arrhythmic compounds on the cardiac action potential: basis for the interpretation of their anti-arrhythmic actions. In: Zipes DP (ed) Progress of cardiology. Lea and Febiger, Philadelphia, pp 37–86
37. Singh BN, Vaughan Williams EM (1970) A third class of antiarrhythmic action. Effects on atrial and ventricular intracellular potentials and other pharmacologic actions on cardiac muscle of in MJ1999 and AH 3474. Br J Pharmacol 39:675–685
38. Singh BN, Vaughan Williams EM (1970) The effect of amiodarone, a new anti-anginal drug, on cardiac muscle. Br J Pharmacol 39:357–367
39. Singh BN, Nademanee K (1985) Control of arrhythmias by selective lengthening of cardiac repolarization: theoretical considerations and clinical observations. Am Heart J 109:421–430
40. Singh BN (ed) (1988) Control of cardiac arrhythmias by lengthening repolarization. Futura, Mount Kisco, pp 1–577
41. Singh BN (1988) When is QT prolongation anti-arrhythmic and when is it pro-arrhythmic? (editorial) Am J Cardiol 63:867–869
42. Singh BN (1989) Controlling cardiac arrhythmias: to delay conduction or to prolong refractoriness? (editorial) Cardiovasc Drugs Therapy 3:671–674
43. Packer M, Lee WH, Kessler PD, Gottlieb SS, Bernstein JL, Kukin ML (1987) Role of neurohumoral mechanisms in determining survival in patients with severe chronic heart failure. Circulation 75 [Suppl IV]:30–35

44. Cardiac Arrhythmia Suppression Trial (CAST) Investigators (1981) Preliminary report: effect of encainide and flecainide on mortality in a randomized trial of arrhythmia suppression after myocardial infarction. N Engl J Med 321:375–385
45. McKenna WJ, Oakley CM, Krikler DM, Goodwin JF (1985) Improved survival with amiodarone in patients with hypertrophic cardiomyopathy and ventricular tachycardia. Br Heart J 53:412–416
46. Burkart F, Pfisterer, Kiowski W, Burckhardt D, Follath F (1989) Improved survival of patients with asymptomatic ventricular arrhythmias after myocardial infarction with amiodarone: a randomized control trial. Circulation 80:11–119
47. Nademanee K, Stevenson W, Weiss J, Singh BN (1988) The role of amiodarone in the survivors of sudden arrhythmic deaths. In: Singh BN (ed) Control of cardiac arrhythmias by lengthening repolarization. Futura, Mount Kisco, pp 489–508
48. Chew CYC, Collett JT, Campbell C, Kannan R, Singh BN (1982) Beneficial effects of amiodarone pretreatment on early ischemic ventricular arrhythmias relative to infarct size and regional myocardial blood flow in the conscious dog. J Cardiovasc Pharmacol 4:1028–1036
49. Patterson E, Eller BT, Abrams GD, Luchessi BR (1983) Ventricular fibrillation in conscious canine preparation of sudden coronary death: prevention by short-term and long-term amiodarone administration. Circulation 68:857–866
50. Takanaka C, Singh BN (1990) Barium-induced non-driven action potentials as a model of triggered automaticity and early afterdepolarizations: differing effects of amiodarone and quinidine and significance of slow-channel activity. J Am Coll Cardiol 15 (1):213–221

Subject Index

AII, cardiac 35
– –, renal 35
– –, vascular 35
ablation, arrhythmogenic substrate 121
–, chemical 104
–, cryoablation 104
–, cryothermal 122
–, direct current shocks 126
–, electrical 104, 108
–, ethanol 108
–, laser 122
–, right atrioventricular junctional 127
–, surgical 123
ACE (angiotensin-converting enzyme) inhibition 25, 33, 36, 39, 66,
"ACE inhibition" 67, 71, 111, 113, 117, 149
action potential, prolongation 21
afterdepolarization, early 20, 21
–, delayed 20, 21
alpha-blockers 149
ambulatory electrocardiographic monitoring 108, 119
amiodarone 108, 115, 116, 136, 166, 168
AMP, cyclic 78
amrinone 78
aneurysm, ventricular 124
aneurysmectomy, ventricular 122
angiotensin-II 55
angiotensin-converting enzyme (see ACE inhibition)
angiotensinogen mRNA 38
animal models for heart failure 20
ANP (atrial natriuretic peptide) 28, 29, 86
– concentrations 28
– levels 28
–, plasma 28
– system 29
–, tissue 28
antiarrhythmic approach 89ff.
antiarrhythmic drugs 16, 17, 29, 91, 92, 102, 105, 108, 111, 113, 138, 168
– therapy 108, 128, 170
antitachycardia function 117
– pacing 96

aortic banding 37
– constriction, experimental 58
– stenosis 57
argon laser 123
arrhythmia(s) 70
–, asymptomatic ventricular arrhythmias 98
–, complex 16
–, malignant 115
–, reentrant 102
–, symptoms 104
–, ventricular 5, 85, 148
–, –, asymptomatic 157
arrhythmogenic effects 167
– factors 16
– substrate 121, 123
– –, ablation 121
arterial hypertension 57
artery disease, coronary 4, 117, 124
ATP 10
ATPase, cardiac myosin 12
atrial fibrillation 102, 105, 127
– natriuretic factor 157
– – peptide (see ANP)
automaticity, abnormal 19, 100
AV nodal tachycardia 105

beta-blockers 149, 164, 166
beta-receptor antagonists 116
biphasic waveform shocks 132

CA^{++} 9
calcium channel blocker 62
calciumantagonists 116
CAMIAT trial 92
CAPS (cardiac arrhythmia pilot study) 138
cardiac AII 35
– arrest 120
– death, sudden cardiac death 3
– dilatation 39
– failure 170
– hypertrophy and dilatation 39
– myocytes 31
– myosin ATPase 12
– RAS 36
– transplantation 163

Subject Index

cardiomyopathy, dilated 6, 24, 119, 123, 161, 164
–, hypertrophic 119, 123, 168
–, tachycardia-related 102
cardioversion, catheter 129
cardioverter/defibrillator, implantable 91, 96, 120
–/–, internal 137
CAST (cardiac arrhythmia suppression) trial 7, 86, 92, 93, 108, 111, 113
"CAST study" 119, 138, 156, 165, 169
catecholamine levels, endogenous 4
catecholamines 20, 31, 113, 148, 167
catheter cardioversion 129
–, electrode 125
cellular hypertrophy 8
chemical ablation 104
cilazapril 111
cilazaprilate 112
circulatory collaps 66
circus-movement tachycardia 103, 105, 108
clinical trial 153
collagen, fibrillar 58
– network, fibrillar 53
– – remodeling 54
– volume fraction 60
compartments, nonmyocyte, remodeling 55
compensated heart failure 33
complex arrhythmias 16
conduction, slowing of 166
congestive heart failure 8, 13, 124
CONSENSUS study 27, 70, 83, 87, 151
contractile proteins 9
contractility abnormalities 53
contraction 9
coronary artery disease 4, 117, 124
– – flow 24
cryoablation 104
cryothermal ablation 122
cyclic AMP 78

d-sotalol 115, 116
death, arrhythmic 156
–, sudden death 3, 43, 91, 98, 106, 113, 119, 136, 138, 140, 164, 169, 170
–, – –, mechanism 162
defibrillation threshold 128
defibrillator, implantable 117
–, –, cardioverter/defibrillator 91, 96, 120, 128, 163
delayed potentials 48
depolarization, afterdepolarization, delayed 20, 21
–, –, early 20, 21
diastolic abnormalities 69
– ventricular function 61
digitalis 113

dilated cardiomyopathy 6, 24, 123, 161, 164
dilatation, left ventricular 11
dilatation, cardiac 39
disopyramide 116
dispersion of refractoriness 19
diuretic drugs/diuretics 101, 113
drug therapy, antiarrhythmic 102, 136
drugs, antiarrhythmic 16, 17, 29, 91, 92, 105, 108, 111, 113, 138, 168
–, diuretic 101
–, positive inotropic drugs 76
dysplasia, right ventricular 108, 122

effect, hemodynamic 113
–, negative inotropic 108
–, proarrhythmic 17, 108, 109, 113, 120, 169
effective refractory period 112, 113
ejection fraction 84, 105, 140, 155
– –, left ventricular 5, 7, 53, 116, 139, 155
electrical ablation 104, 108
– instability 101
electrocardiographic monitoring, ambulatory 108, 119
electrode arrays, multiple 122
– catheters 125
– configuration 129
–, patch 130
electrogram, intracardiac 115
–, surface 115
electrolyte abnormalities 86
electrophysiological parameters 112
– testing 43
EMIAT trial 92
enalapril 157
encainide 108, 140, 165, 166
endocardial recordings 121
– resection 104
endogenous catecholamine levels 4
energy starvation 13
– –, chronic 12
enzyme, angiotensin converting enzyme inhibitor 66
epicardial recordings 121
ethanol ablation 108
excitability, recovery of 19
exercise capacity 53
experimental aortic constriction 58
– heart failure 37, 39
– hypertension 61

fibrillar collagen 58
– – network 53
fibrillation, atrial 102, 105, 127
– threshold, ventricular 4
–, ventricular 17, 106, 113, 120, 162

Subject Index

fibrosis, interstitial 24, 58, 60
–, myocardial 57, 61
flecainide 95, 108, 115, 116, 139, 140, 165, 166

gene expression 12
growth factors 31

heart disease, valvular 119
– failure 162
– –, acute 66
– –, chronic 66
– –, compensated 33
– –, congestive 13, 124
– –, experimental 37, 39
– –, unstable 79
– hypertrophy 19
hemodynamic approach 51ff.
– effect 113
Holter recording/monitoring 92, 111, 113, 162, 168
human myocardium 57
hypertension, arterial 57
–, experimental 61
–, renovascular (RHT) 61
hypertensive rats, spontaneously 36
hypertrophic cardiomyopathy 123, 168
hypertrophied myocardium 55
hypertrophy 19, 21
– and dilatation, cardiac 39
–, early, left ventricular dilatation 11
– of myocytes 24
–, regression of 72
hypokalemia 86, 127, 167
hypomagnesemia 127, 167

impaired left ventricular function 16
implantable cardioverter/defibrillator 91, 96, 117, 120, 128, 163
    see defibrillator and cardioverter
inducible ventricular tachycardia 48
infarction, myocardial 106, 124
–, –, acute 5
–, postmyocardial 5
–, – infarction period 111
inotropic agents 85, 149
– drugs, positive 76
– effects, negative 102
internal cardioverter/defibrillator 137
interstitial fibrosis 24, 58, 60
intracardiac electrogram 115
intraoperative ventricular mapping 122
ischemic area 19

Langendorf perfused rings 105
– preparation 37
laser ablation 122
–, argon 123

late potentials 43, 44
left ventricular dilatation 11
– – dysfunction 3, 5, 76, 120, 139, 157
– – ejection 124
– – – fraction 5, 7, 53, 116, 139, 155
– – function 24, 46, 113, 122
– – –, diastolic 61
– – –, impaired 16
– – –, systolic 61
– – hypertrophy 3, 54
– – – early hypertrophy 11
lidocaine 116
life, quality of 147

malignant arrhythmias 115
– ventricular tachyarrhythmias, nonpharmacologic therapy 119
map-guided surgery 121
mapping 124
– techniques 121
–, ventricular, intraoperative 122
mexiletine 115, 116
MILIS trial 5
monitoring, electrocardiographic, ambulatory 108, 119
–, Holter recording/monitoring 92, 111, 113, 162, 168
moricizine 140
mortality 5, 117, 151, 154, 161, 166–168
–, perioperative 122, 128
– rate 147, 148
MPIP study 5
mRNA, angiotensinogen 38
–, renin 38
muscle blood flow, skeletal 70
myocardial fibrosis 57, 61
– function 83, 84
– hypertrophy 9
– infarction 106, 124
– –, acute 5
– proteins 12
– stiffness 54
myocardium, human 57
–, hypertrophied 55
–, stunned 77
myocytes, cardiac 31
–, hypertrophy of 24
myosin 12
– ATPase, cardiac 12

Na^+-H^+ exchange 38
Na^+/Ca^{++} exchanger 10
natriuretic factor, atrial 157
negative inotropic effect 108
nervous system, sympathetic 86, 100, 101
neuroendocrine activation 83
neurohormonal control mechanism 33

neurohormones, plasma 33
nifedipine 62
nonmyocyte compartments, remodeling 55
nonpharmacologic therapy 128
– – for malignant ventricular tachyarrhythmias 119
nonsustained ventricular tachycardia 44, 119, 138, 162, 168
norepinephrine 157

overdrive pacing 115
– stimulation 102

pacing, antitachycardia 96
–, overdrive 115
patch electrodes 130
perioperative mortality 122, 128
peripheral vascular resistance 70
phosphates, high-energy 9
phosphodiesterase (PDE) inhibitors 101, 113
phosphodiesterase-III inhibitors 78
placebo control 151
plasma ANP 28
– neurohormones 33
– renin activity 39
positive inotropic drugs 76
postmyocardial infarction period 111
potassium-channel blockers 166
potential(s), delayed 48
–, late 43, 44
–, proarrhythmic 102
pressure-overload ventricles 20
proarrhythmic effect 17, 108, 109, 113, 120, 169
– potential 102
procainamide 116, 136
prognosis 53, 83, 102, 104, 106, 117, 145ff.
prognostic factors 156
– indices 83
– significance 46
programmed stimulation 43
prolongation of action potential 21
PROMISE (prospective randomized milrinone survival evaluation) 159
propafenone 115, 116
proteins, contractile 9
–, myocardial 12
–, regulatory 81
pulsed laser lesion 123
pump function 13, 104

quality of life 147
quinidine 115, 116, 136

randomized controlled study 148
– trial(s) 150, 159

RAS (renin-angiotensin system) 33ff., 101, 167
–, cardiac 36
–, renal 38
–, tissue 33, 34
–, vascular 35
rats, spontaneously hypertensive 36
receptor population 81
recordings, endocardial 121
–, epicardial 121
recovery of excitability 19
reentrant arrhythmias 102
reentry, circuit 114
–, depolarizations 21
–, double-wave 105, 106
–, single-wave 105
–, substrates for 17
–, triggers for 19
refractoriness, dispersion of 19
refractory period, effective 112, 113
regional wall motion stress 113
regression of hypertrophy 72
regulatory proteins 81
relaxation 9
remodeling of nonmyocyte compartments 55
renal AII 35
– RAS 38
renin activity, plasma 39
– mRNA 38
renin-angiotensin system (see RAS)
renovascular hypertension (RHT) 61
repolarization 112
resection, endocardial 104
–, subendocardial 120, 122
reticulum, sarcoplasmic 9, 10
rhythm disturbances 43
right ventricular dysplasia 108, 122
risk factors 5
RNA (see also mRNA) 38

sarcoplasmic reticulum 9, 10
SAVE (study to avoid ventricular enlargement) 158
skeletal muscle blood flow 70
SOLVD (studies of left ventricular dysfunction) 157
sotalol 116
–, d-sotalol 115, 116
spontaneously hypertensive rats 36
stiffness 60
stimulation, programmed 43
stone heart 11
stunned myocardium 77
subendocardial resection 120, 122
sudden death 43, 91, 98, 106, 113, 119, 136, 138, 140, 164, 169, 170
– –, mechanism 162

Subject Index

supraventricular tachycardia 105
surface electrogram 115
surgery, map-guided 121
surgical ablation 123
survival 147
sustained tachycardia 104
– ventricular tachycardia 44, 112, 113, 120, 124
sympathetic nervous system 86, 100, 101
– outflow 16
– overactivity 27
– withdrawal 27
systolic function 69
– ventricular function 61

tachyarrhythmias, ventricular, origin of 121
tachycardia, AV nodal 105
–, circus-movement 103, 105, 108
–, origin of 104
–, recurrant ventricular tachycardia 96
–, supraventricular 105
–, sustained 104
–, ventricular 7, 47, 102, 105, 106, 136, 148, 162
–, –, idiopathic VT 106
–, –, inducible 48
–, –, nonsustained VT 44, 106, 119, 138, 162, 168
–, –, sustained VT 44, 106, 112, 113, 120, 124
–, ventricular, VT acceleration 106
tachycardia-related cardiomyopathy 102
therapy, antiarrhythmic 128, 170
–, nonpharmacologic 119
–, vasodilator 161
tissue ANP 28
– renin-angiotensin system 33
torsades de pointes 102, 167
transplantation, cardiac 163
triggered activity 17, 19, 100
– automaticity 4

valvular heart disease 6, 119
vascular AII 35
– resistance, peripheral 70
vasodilator(s) 66, 68
– therapy 161

vasopressor systems 25
ventricles, pressure-overload 20
ventricular aneurysm 124
– aneurysmectomy 122
– arrhythmia(s) 5, 85, 148
– –, asymptomatic 98, 161
– dilatation, left, and early hypertrophy 11
– dysfunction 140
– –, left 3, 5, 76, 120, 139, 157
– dysplasia, right 108, 122
– ectopic activity, complex 164
– ejection 162
– – fraction, left 5, 7, 53, 116, 124, 139, 155
– fibrillation 17, 106, 113, 120, 162
– – threshold 4
– function, left 24, 46, 122
– –, –, diastolic 61
– –, –, impaired 16
– –, –, systolic 61
– hypertrophy, left 3, 54
– mapping, intraoperative 122
– rhythm disturbances 43
– stimulation, programmed 137, 138
– tachyarrhythmias, malignant, nonpharmacologic therapy 119
– –, origin of 121
– tachycardia 7, 47, 102, 105, 106, 136, 148, 162
– –, idiopathic VT 106
– –, incessant sustained 123
– –, inducible 48
– –, multiple 125
– –, nonsustained VT 44, 106
– –, pleomorphic 125
– –, recurrant 96
– –, sustained VT 44, 106
– –, VT acceleration 106
– wall stress 24, 148
volume fraction, collagen 60

wall motion stress, regional 113
– stress, ventricular 24, 148
waveform shocks, biphasic 132
Wolff-Parkinson-White syndrome 108

xamoterol 155

J. Brachmann, A. Schömig,
University of Heidelberg (Eds.)

Adrenergic System and Ventricular Arrythmias in Myocardial Infarction

1989. XIII, 363 pp. 126 figs. 14 tabs. Hardcover DM 126,-
ISBN 3-540-50593-8

This book presents new aspects on electrophysiological mechanisms and catecholaminergic contributions in the setting of acute and chronic myocardial ischemia. Special emphasis is placed on the full scope from basic molecular and cellular mechanisms to experimental models of close clinical proximity. A number of internationally distinguished scientists present their latest findings in this significant research area within the perimeter of cardiovascular disease which continues to lead mortality statistics in most industrialized countries.

Contents of this book cover, in addition to other subjects, release and uptake of catecholamines in ischemia, regulation of receptors, adrenergic contribution to ventricular arrhythmias and mechanisms of ischemic malignant arrhythmias as well as underlying changes in membrane currents and the electrophysiological response to beta-adrenergic blocking drugs. In addition to original contributions, a number of editorial chapters are included for conclusions and future development in these areas.

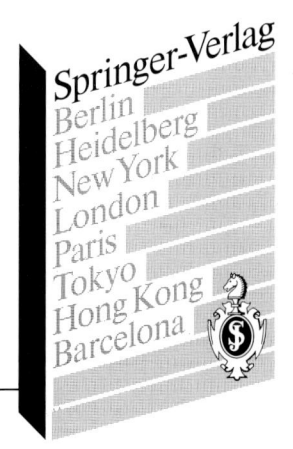

Springer-Verlag
Berlin
Heidelberg
New York
London
Paris
Tokyo
Hong Kong
Barcelona